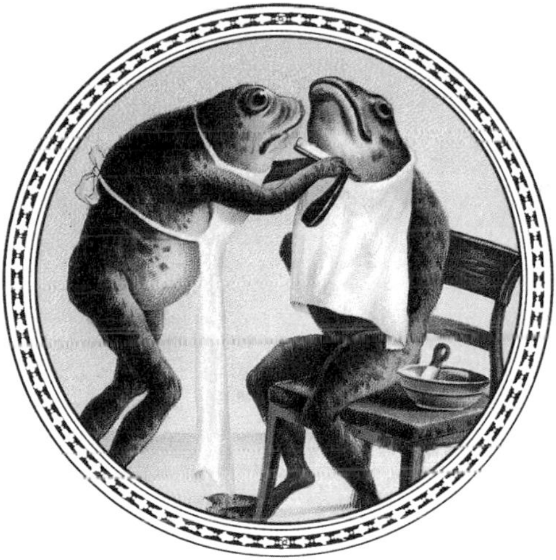

Also by Wallace Pinfold

Rising to the Occasion
with Edith Hazard

A CLOSER SHAVE

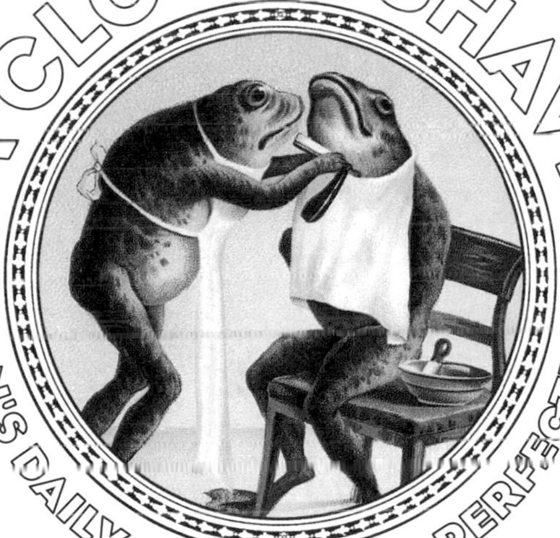

MAN'S DAILY SEARCH FOR PERFECTION

Wallace G. Pinfold

ARTISAN

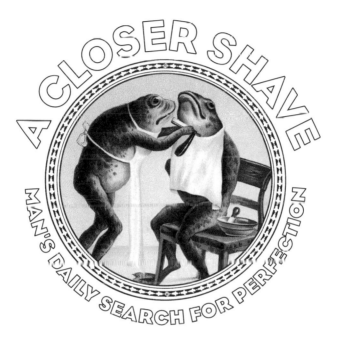

Permissions, constituting a continuation of this copyright page, appear on page 159.

DESIGNER: Pat Tan
PICTURE RESEARCH & EDITING: Alexandra Truitt and Jerry Marshall

Published in 1999 by Artisan,
a division of Workman Publishing Company, Inc.
708 Broadway
New York, N.Y. 10003

Library of Congress Cataloging-in-Publication Data
Pinfold, Wallace.
A closer shave: man's daily search for perfection / Wallace G. Pinfold.
p. cm.
ISBN 1-57965-136-4 (hardcover)
1. Shaving—History. I. Title.
TT964.P56 1999
646.7'24—dc21 98-51400
CIP

Printed in Canada

10 9 8 7 6 5 4 3 2 1

First Printing

For my father

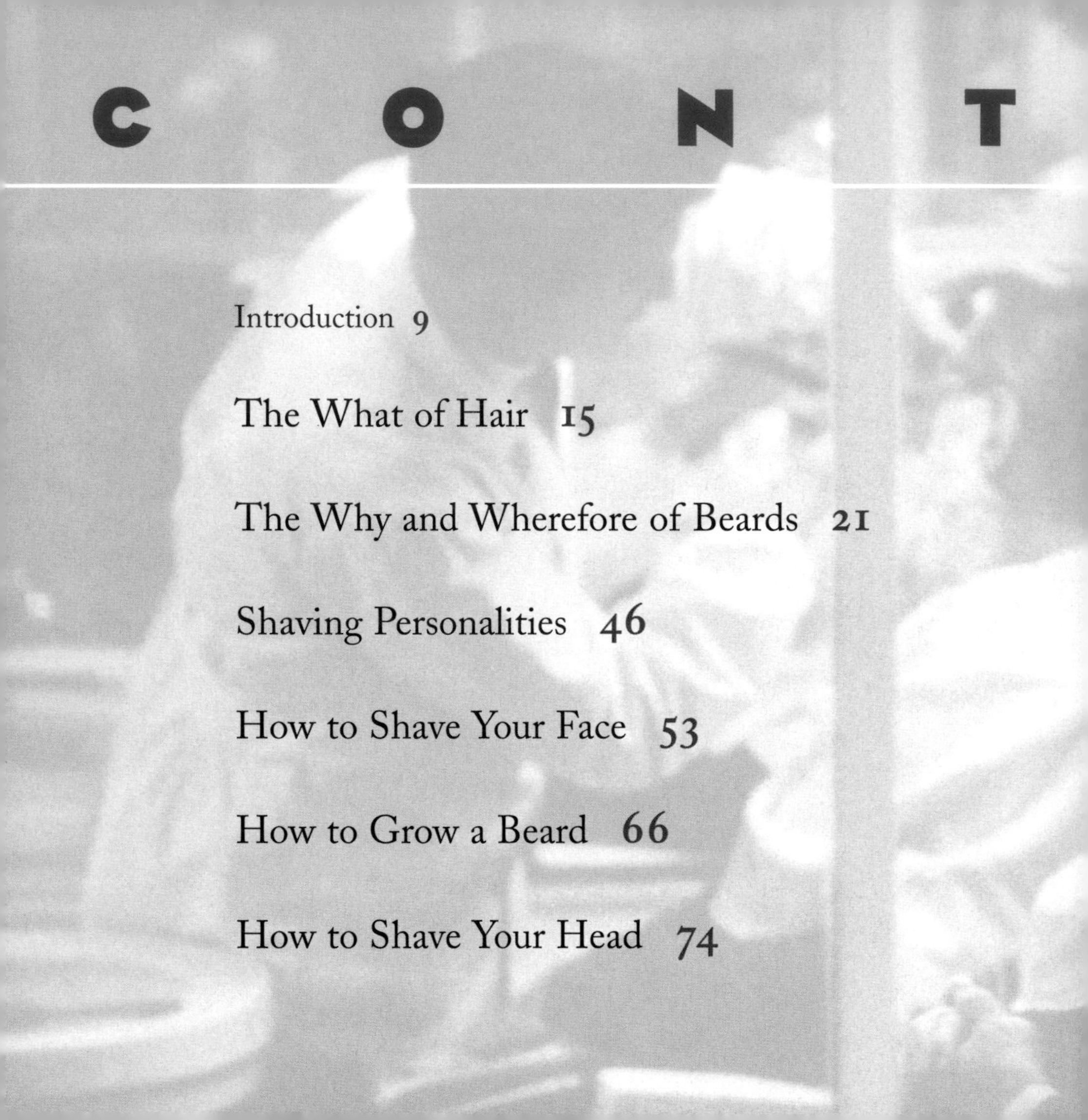

C O N T

Introduction 9

The What of Hair 15

The Why and Wherefore of Beards 21

Shaving Personalities 46

How to Shave Your Face 53

How to Grow a Beard 66

How to Shave Your Head 74

E N T S

Straight Razors
and Barbershop Shaves 81

The March of Progress 96

Edsels and Edisons 111

The Equipment 124

Life's Rich Pattern 143

Acknowledgments 157
Photography and Illustration Credits 158

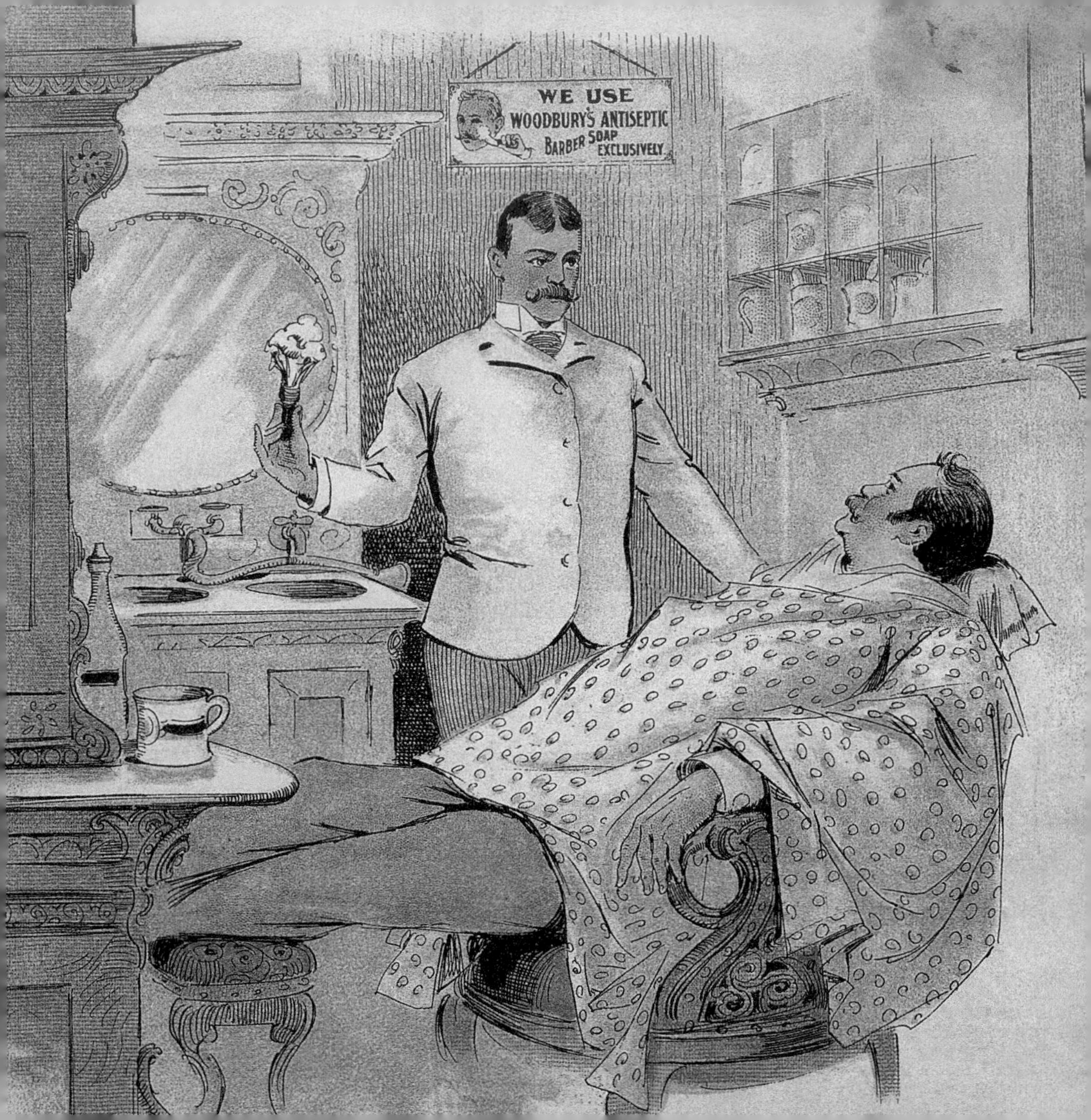
WE USE
WOODBURY'S ANTISEPTIC
BARBER SOAP
EXCLUSIVELY.

INTRODUCTION

I've been bearded and clean-shaven. I've obsessed about the proportions of a mustache and wondered if a little wax wouldn't improve its look. Sometimes having a beard has been a convenience; other times I grew one because I thought it looked good. Once I grew one to look older. But I've been mostly clean-shaven, and like most men over the age of fourteen, have had a relationship with a razor all my adult life.

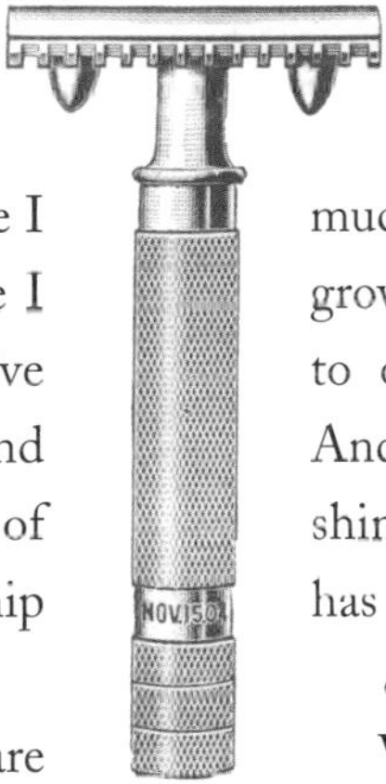

Body hair is a trait we share with other mammals. Great whales, ring-tailed cats, you name it. Our peculiarly human determination to *do* something about this hair is what sets us apart from the rest of the animal kingdom. We assume, for example, that orangutans are content with the way they look. *Homo sapiens,* we know firsthand, never are. Either we have too much or too little hair. It grows where we don't want it to or it doesn't grow at all. And every morning, rain or shine, the male of the species has a beard to contend with.

A beard and an attitude.

What's the use, a man asks himself. While I sleep, my beard is growing. While I'm driving to work or working in the yard, my beard is growing. While I'm reading a book, writing a check, brewing coffee—whatever I'm doing, shadow creeps along my jawline. Even as I'm shaving, my beard continues its inexorable growth.

So why bother? Well, we shave to look good. We shave to please others. We shave, many of us, because at this particular moment in our history, the majority of male citizens are clean-shaven. No sumptuary laws need regulate this because custom and fashion are just as binding as ordinance and statute.

Rather than regarding this daily task as drudgery, we'd do better to enjoy it. More than watching sports, more than checking car prices, more than acting sensitive, shaving is *the* defining male activity. And the daily opportunity to get a good, close shave is as near as most men will get to perfection in this life.

What's more, if a man wants to shave, or must, there's never been a better time in human history to do so. The implements available to our Bronze Age ancestors inspire curiosity and respect. The straight razors that were men's only choice until the first years of the twentieth century inspire respect and *fear*. Thanks to the invention of the safety razor one hundred years ago, shaving instruments are easier to use, more affordable, and less dangerous than ever before. Thanks to the introduction of the electric shaver in 1929, a man can shave anywhere he can find a power source.

The forward march of technology and a broad reading of the

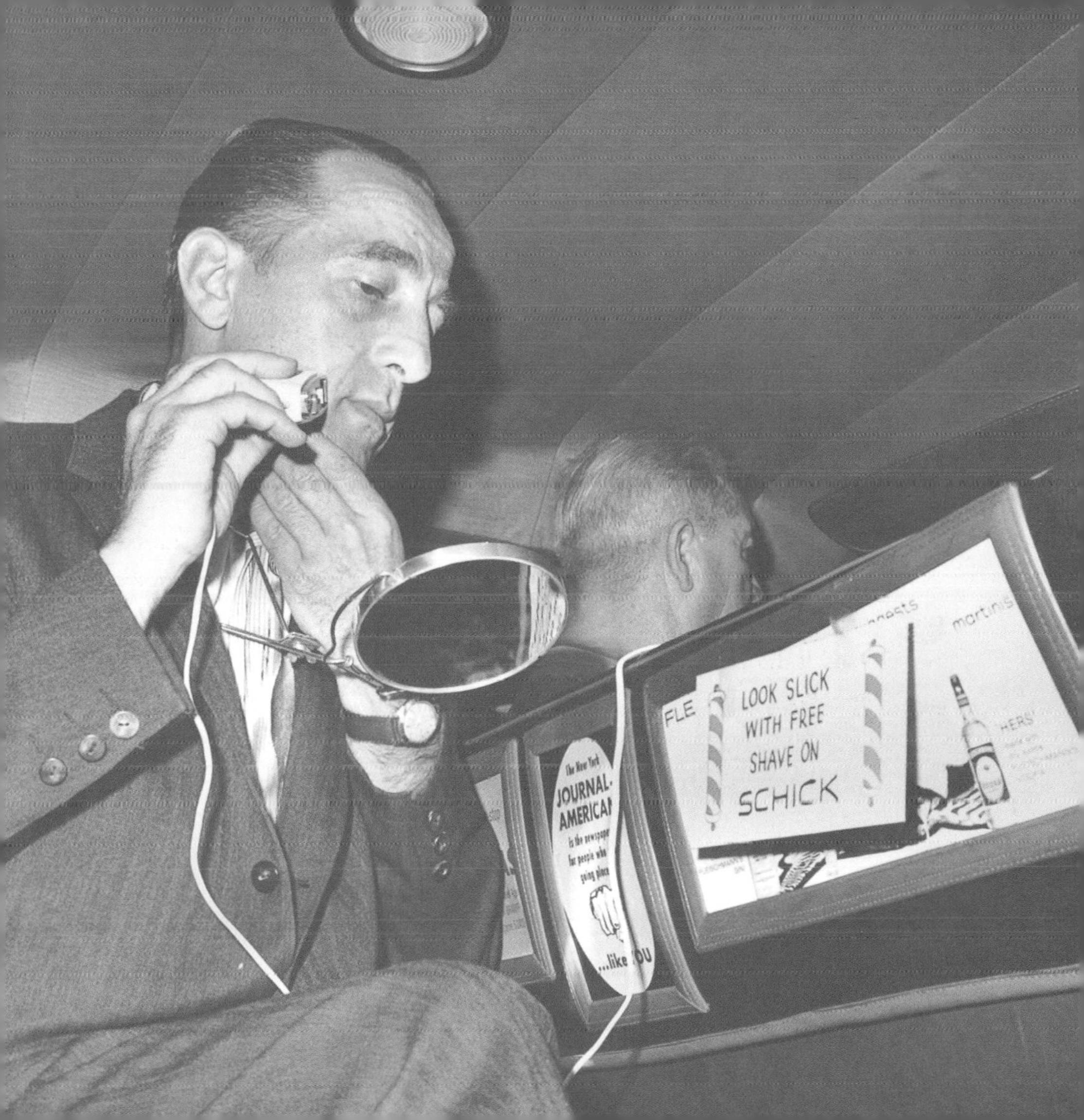
LOOK SLICK
WITH FREE
SHAVE ON
SCHICK
martinis
The New York
JOURNAL-

First Amendment suggest that the question "To shave or not to shave?" has no right answer. And the briefest glance at other times and other cultures makes us appreciate our freedom to decide for ourselves. For example, a conservative interpretation of Islamic law makes it a man's duty to cultivate a beard. A literal reading of Leviticus imposes the same obligation on Jews and Christians alike. Being required to grow a beard is as burdensome as having to shave—both are duties imposed from above.

Where shaving is concerned, we've come a long way. The manliest of manly activities has a heroic past and a present rich with opportunity. What better way to improve the five minutes spent shaving every morning than in reflecting on the activity itself? After all, you're looking at yourself in a mirror. Modify Descartes' motto and make it your own: *Rado ergo sum.*

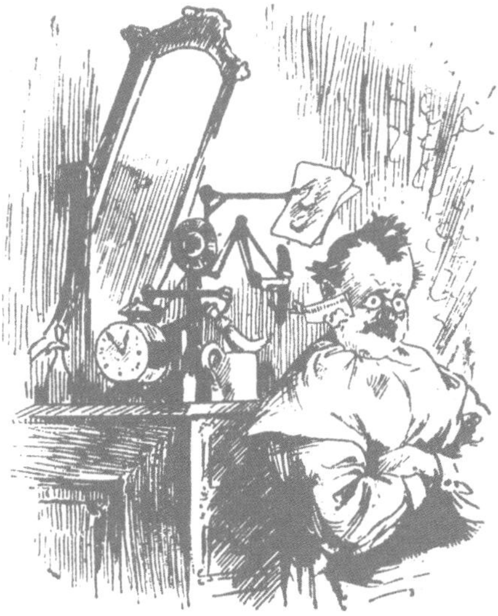

NUBA

In the Kordofan province of the Islamic Democratic Republic of the Sudan, people believe that shaving, hair grooming, and body painting are the activities that distinguish human beings from animals. Young men of the southeastern Nuba group shave bodies, heads, and faces, oil their skins, and, when time permits and occasion requires, paint patterns on their naked selves as beautiful and as graphically dramatic as the best Japanese tattoos. In southeastern Nuba myth, monkeys once spoke the same language as men, so it is not the ability to speak that makes humans human—it is the ability to remove hair.

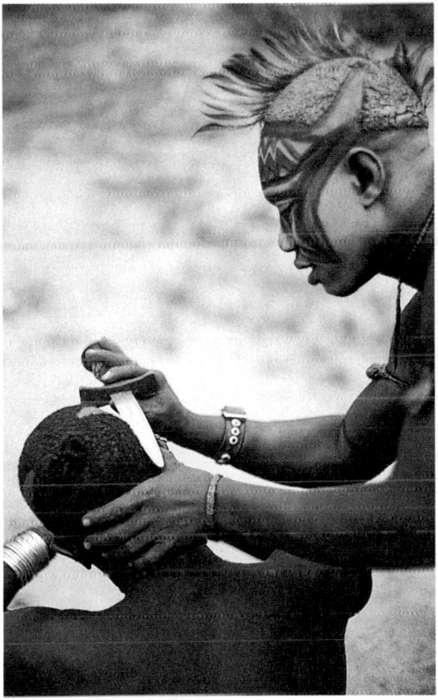

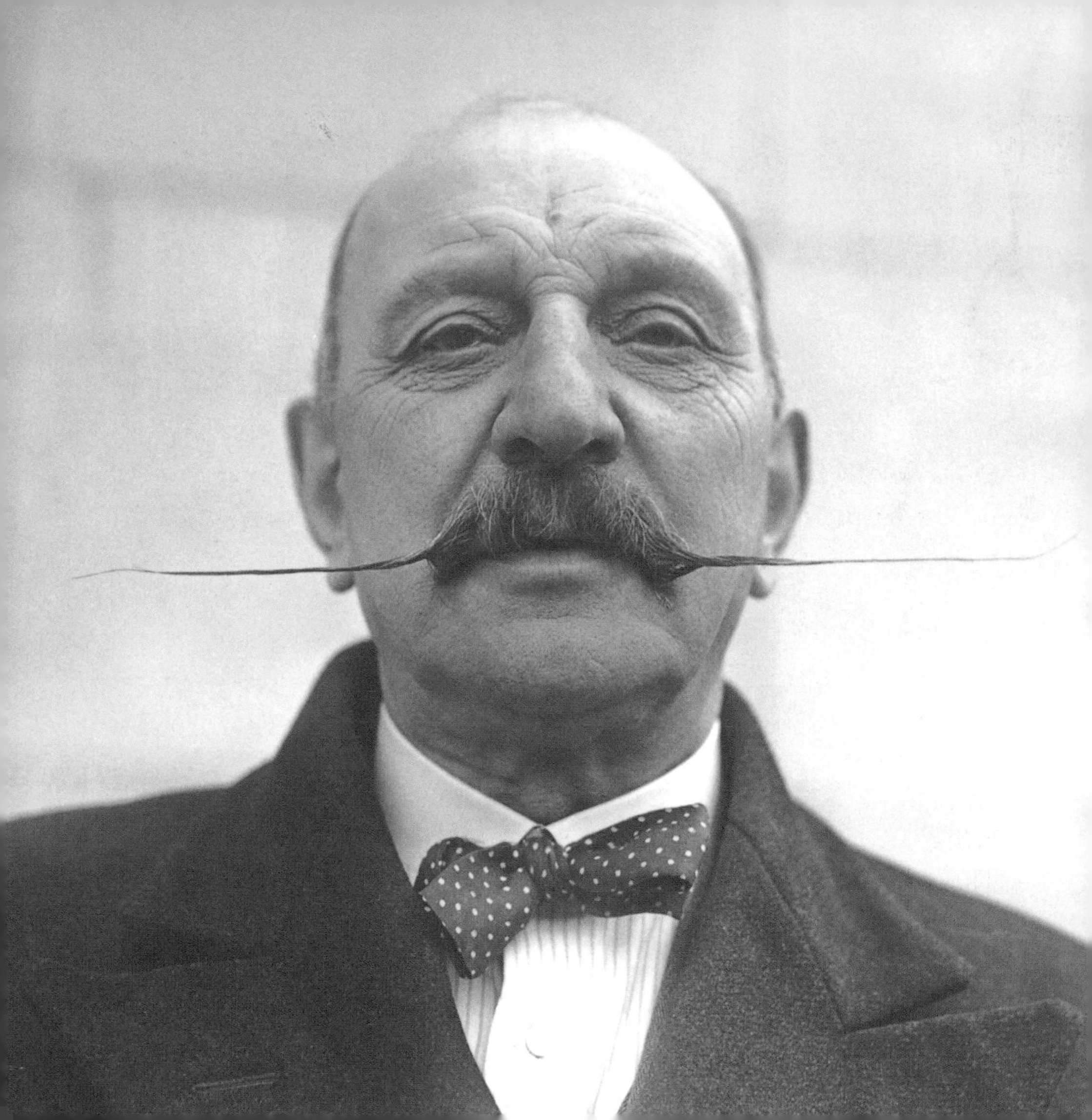

THE WHAT OF HAIR

But the very hairs of your head are all numbered.
Matthew 10:30

Hair. It's the subject of musicals, fairy tales, and so many magazine articles it would take forever to read them. In humans, it grows about .35 millimeters a day (1 centimeter a month, 1 inch every two to three months, as much as 5 or 6 inches a year). It never rests. Some five million follicles cover the human body and each one has its own growth cycle. In the scalp, for instance, a hair grows for three to five years. The growing phase of a hair of the eyebrows, on the other hand, is only about ten weeks and the hairs never grow very long. We have no synchronized and seasonal waves of hair growth and shedding as some animals do, although those of us living in the north Temperate Zone, curiously, shed more hairs in November than in any other month.

All hair is not alike. Some of the hair on our bodies and all of the hair on our heads and beards—is pigmented. Then there's the nearly invisible stuff that covers the rest of the body and is not. We're less hairy than gibbons and gorillas, but we have three times more hair than chimpanzees do. But because chimps have longer, coarser hair than ours, we look naked by comparison.

The number of hair follicles per square inch of face determines the kind of beard a man has. If the distribution of beard hair were uniform over the face, we'd all look like Wookies. Instead, the lower part of the cheeks has the lowest concentration of hair follicles, the upper lip the highest. This is why more men can grow satisfactory mustaches than satisfactory beards.

The kind of beard a man has and the frequency with which he has to shave have a racial component. Baldly stated, some races are hairier than others. Caucasians—people from Europe and the Middle East—are the hairiest, Asians the least hairy, and Africans fall somewhere in between. Among Caucasoids, the greatest development of beard and body hair is seen on males from the eastern Mediterranean and the Near East.

Just for the record and while we're on the subject, in different races, beards reach their full potential at different rates. A comparison of Caucasoid and Asian men of different ages shows that among the former, beards are at their thickest (showing the greatest number of hairs per square inch) by the time a man is thirty-five. It will be another thirty years before a Chinese man's chin has reached its full potential.

What do all these facts about beard biology mean? Simply this: A man's ability to grow a beard or mustache worthy of a place in the *Guinness Book of World Records* has nothing to do with a positive attitude or superior virility. It has

You may lament how coarse your beard is and the fact that you have to shave two times a day. But consider the lot of Superman:

"Any attempt to cut Superman's hair by ordinary means results only in the shattering of whatever scissors are being used, but Superman can cut his own hair when absolutely necessary by subjecting it to the concentrated power of his X-Ray vision. In a red-sun environment, however, where Superman has no superpowers, his hair loses its indestructibility and begins to grow. If he undertakes a mission to such a planet, it is best for him to shave and trim his hair before returning to the yellow-sun environment of Earth, where his hair will once again become indestructible."

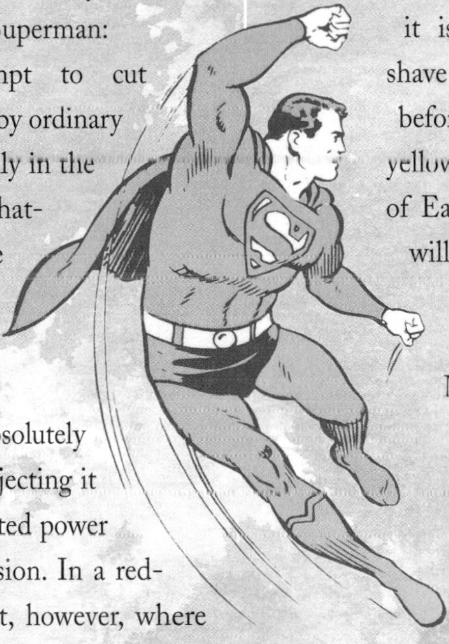

Michael L. Fleisher,
The Great Superman Book

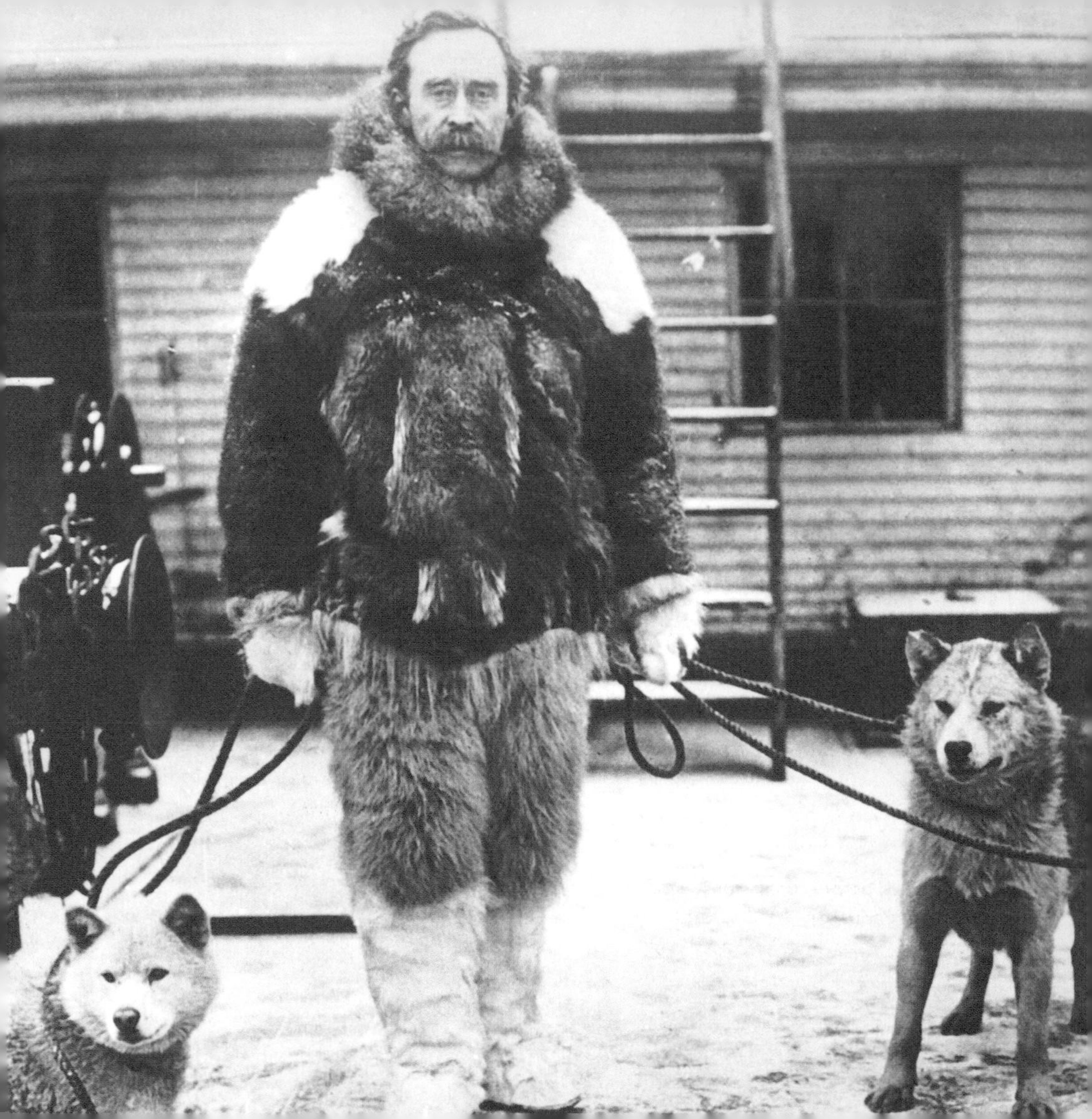

everything to do with the accidents of world history—in other words, his genetic baggage.

Growth After Death

The belief that the beard—as well as the hair, fingernails, and toenails—continues to grow after death has been around at least since the time of the Romans. Although it's completely untrue, it's perfectly understandable. After death, tissues and muscles dry and contract, creating the illusion that the nails and hair have grown, simply because more of each material is exposed.

Left: Human beings, unlike their sled dogs, can't adapt to extreme cold by growing more hair. Admiral Peary donned a fur suit—and grew a mustache.

Moreover, hair and nails do not deteriorate as quickly as the body's other tissues.

After death, the fluid contents of the skull slowly evaporate, making the hair look as if it is "standing up." For the same reason, a dead man's whiskers may seem to grow, and a scrupulous undertaker may shave a corpse more than once before the funeral. But it's not a new beard that has grown; it's simply the old one that has been more exposed.

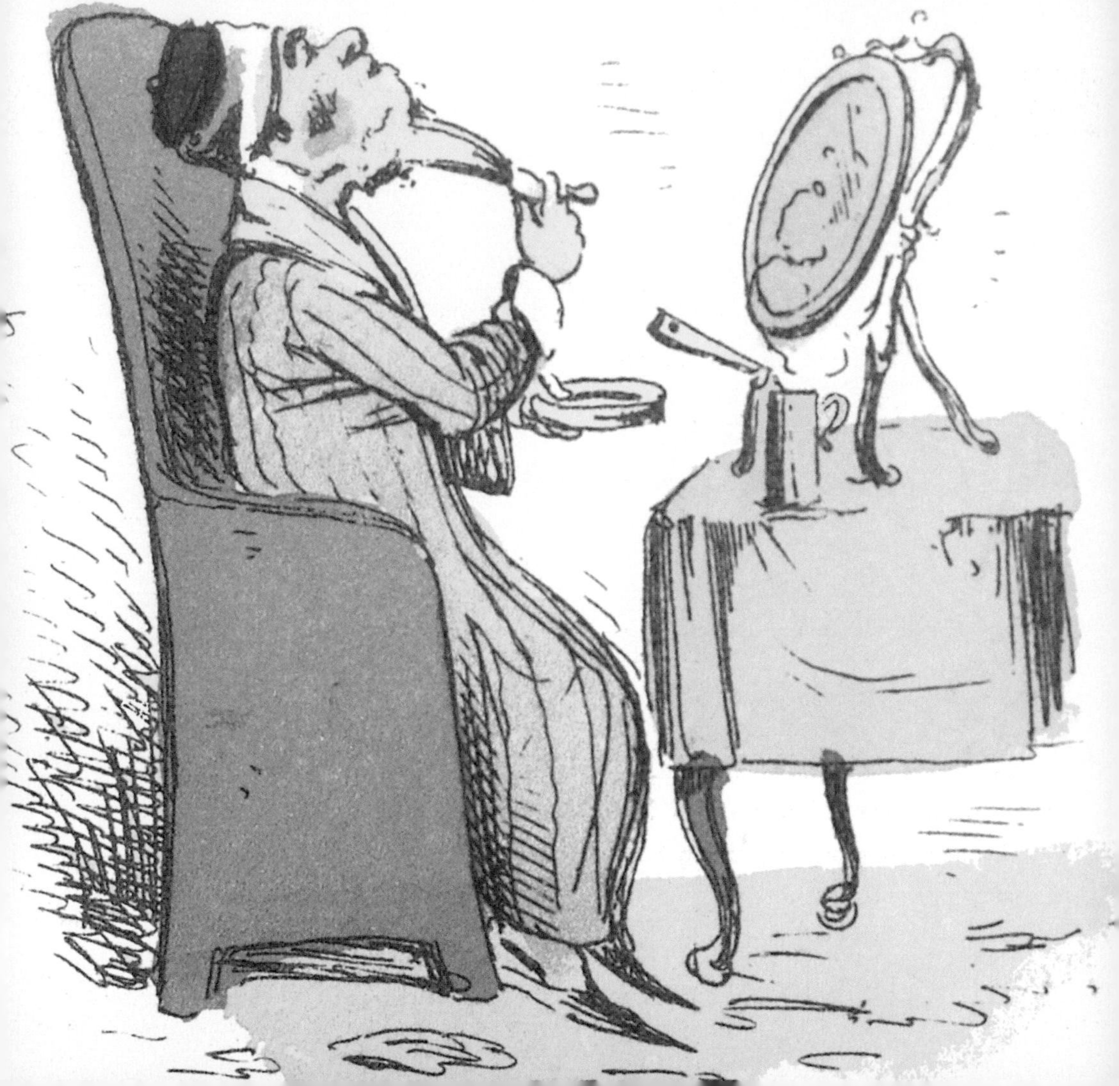

THE WHY AND WHEREFORE OF BEARDS

Throughout history, each feature of facial hair [has] had its own significance and how a man . . . shaved his beard is an indication of how he saw himself and how he was regarded by others.

Giles Constable, Introduction to *Apologia de Barbis*

Why is it that most mornings of your adult life you don't feel quite right about facing the day until you've shaved? You feel grubby, unclean, unfit for human society. You may like shaving; you may hate shaving, its dailiness may bore you silly, but for all kinds of reasons you'll do it as long as you have the strength to press the button on your can of Barbasol.

We consider our decision to shave or not to shave an individual decision. In fact, we're only part right. The decision to shave or let one's beard grow carries a social message and the message changes over time.

Egyptian Shavers

In ancient Egypt, full beards and overall hairiness represented uncleanliness and negligence. In tomb paintings and reliefs, only foreigners and people from the lowest classes of society are represented as having any kind of body hair. The earliest Egyptians may have worn their hair long and wavy, decorated with an ostrich feather, but by the time bronze had replaced copper in the manufacture of razors, natural hair was cropped as short as possible, and men and women donned wigs for public occasions. A man might wear a thin

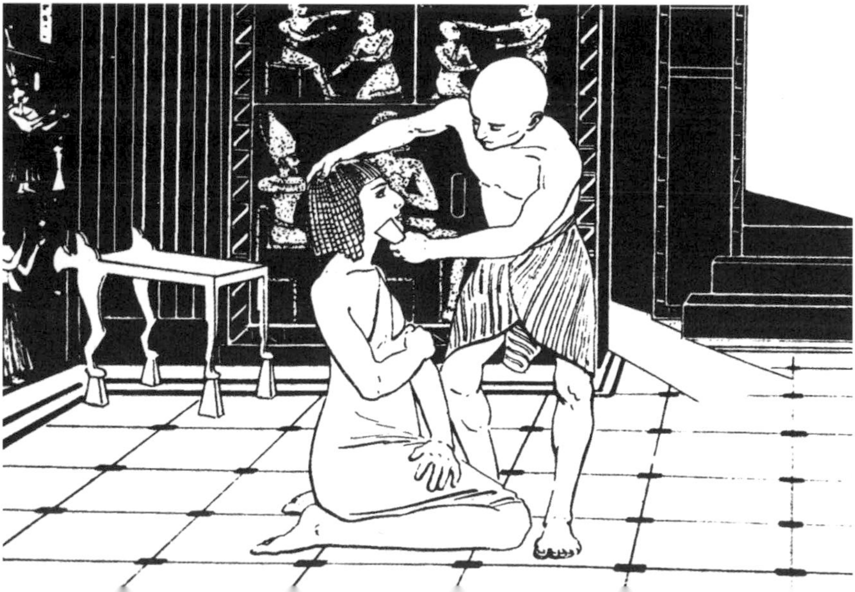

mustache or a short, neatly trimmed beard, but in general the shaved head and body were the norm. It was only in special circumstances, in times of mourning, for instance, that facial stubble was allowed.

Artisans with special tonsorial skills, called *chaku* (shavers), were employed by royal and noble households, temples, and, so it seems, the army. Other shavers served the general populace, but given the artifacts found by archaeologists, it seems likely that routine shaving and depilation were done by people in their homes. Wealthier people used razors, knives, and tweezers made of copper and bronze; the poor made do with knives and scrapers made of flint.

For all this desire to be clean-shaven all over, Egyptian royalty, men and women alike, wore a metal false beard or postiche, held in place by a ribbon tied over the head and attached with a gold chin strap, a custom that went back to the Early Dynastic Period.

Alexander the Great

Until Alexander the Great (356–323 B.C.) commanded his soldiers to shave their beards, the custom was practically unknown. (The Greek historian Herodotus, writing a century before Alexander's time, described the smooth faced Egyptians' repulsion for the hairy Greeks.) The reasons were practical: In hand-to-hand combat, beards served as "handles" for the enemy to grab. Alexander being beardless may have been inspired by his desire to more closely resemble the god Apollo, eternally young, but whatever the reason, Alexander's clean-shaven face inaugurated a long period of beardlessness in the Greco-Roman world.

Hadrian

In the early days of the Empire, Roman leaders were clean-shaven. The emperor Hadrian (A.D. 117–38) completed the Parthenon, built a wall across Britain, and for a time revived the fashion for beards. Known in his time as a reformer and a patron of learning and the arts, the emperor was not a handsome man. He bore ugly battle scars on his face and had a wart on his chin. Hadrian grew a beard to hide these defects hoping to make a better impression on his subjects when he traveled around the Empire.

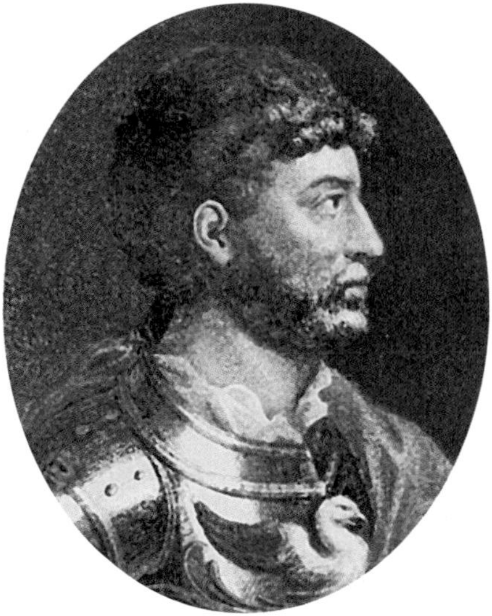

Above: Hadrian, Roman emperor (A.D. 117–38)

CROWNED HEADS

The fashion for beards has waxed and waned throughout history. When kings still counted and beards were in fashion, kings set the style for beards.

At the time of the Norman Conquest (1066), whiskers were not worn in England. William the Conqueror and his soldiers were mostly clean-shaven and the merest mustache made a man conspicuous. But fashions change and it wasn't long before Bishop Serle was drawing unflattering parallels between the men of the Normanized English court and "filthy goats and bristly Saracens."

During his reign, Henry II (1154–89) was clean-shaven; Henry III (1216–72) had a long full beard; Edward II (1307–27) wore his whiskers in three great ringlets; Edward III (1327–77) affected a well-kept forked beard. Richard II (1377–99) wore a little tuft on either side of his chin; Henry IV (1399–1413) also sported tufts and curled them.

By the time Henry VIII (1509–47) came to the throne, beards had been out of fashion for some time. According to the borough records of Canterbury, citizens paid a penalty for wearing beards, and lawyers with long beards wishing to sit at the great table at Lincoln's Inn (the law courts) were charged double fees. In 1535, Henry ordered his courtiers to "poll their hair" and permit a crisp beard to grow. His daughter Elizabeth (1558–1603) sent four

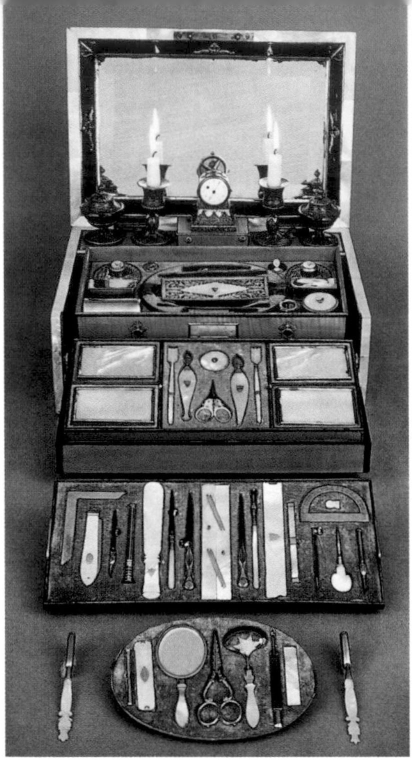

Above: This fine steel and mother-of-pearl traveling kit kept nineteenth-century King Ferdinand VII of Spain well-trimmed and barbered.

bearded men to Moscow as her envoys. One of them, George Kenilworth, boasted whiskers so long—five feet twenty-one inches from tip to chin—that Ivan the Terrible, not known for his good humor, was so delighted with the beard he burst out laughing and couldn't resist playing with it.

Henry VIII's French contemporary, Francis I (1515–47), once, in a snowball fight, suffered a head wound serious enough to require that his scalp be shaved. While the king recuperated, his face went unshaved. By the time he was fit to be seen by his subjects, he had a handsome beard and short hair. As a result, short hair became fashionable and courtiers began to let their beards grow. In a miniature depicting Francis I's son, Henry II, healing the scrofulous the year he became king, he wears his hair and beard the way his father did.

Samuel Pepys

Samuel Pepys (1633–1703) in his diary wrote a testimonial to the pleasures of a daily shave. Always game, the diarist of the Great Fire

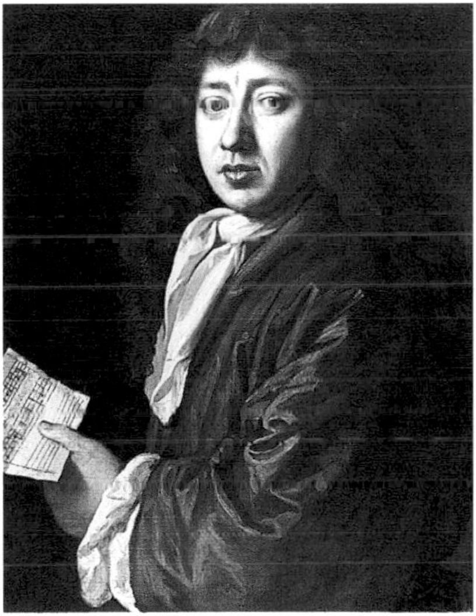

Above: "Lord! How ugly I was yesterday and how fine today," wrote Pepys after shaving off a week's worth of stubble.

of London tried rubbing his beard away with a pumice stone, a technique used a millennium and more before by Roman legionnaires. Later, he learned how to use the straight razor and was pleased by the savings in time, money, and blood thereby achieved. Intending to work at home one day, Pepys writes that he went into his study unshaven but that "without being shaved I am not fully awake nor ready to settle to business."

Peter the Great

Death and taxes, we are tirelessly told, are inescapable. So are opinions about beards.

Peter the Great of Russia (1672–1725) is known for his colossal

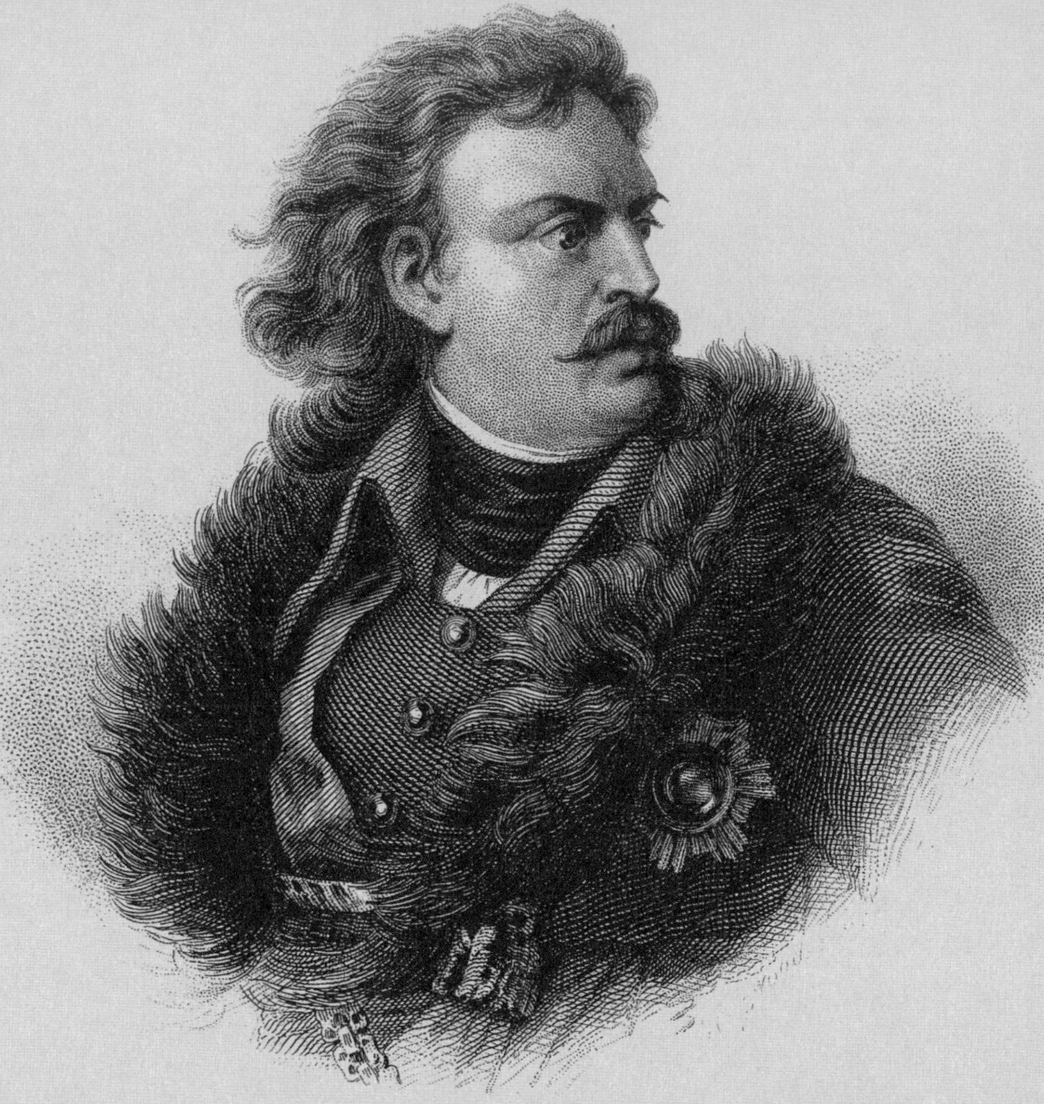

stature—six feet seven—his heavy drinking, and his great cruelty. He founded St. Petersburg, created the Russian fleet, and modernized Russia. In 1705, as part of his campaign to Westernize his empire, he began requiring his subjects to shave their beards. Russians who refused were required to pay a beard tax. This outlawing of beards might seem like aesthetic quirkiness to a modern reader; however, to Peter's subjects it was a major insult to Russian tradition. According to Peter's predecessor, Ivan the Terrible, "To shave the beard is a sin that the blood of all the martyrs cannot cleanse."

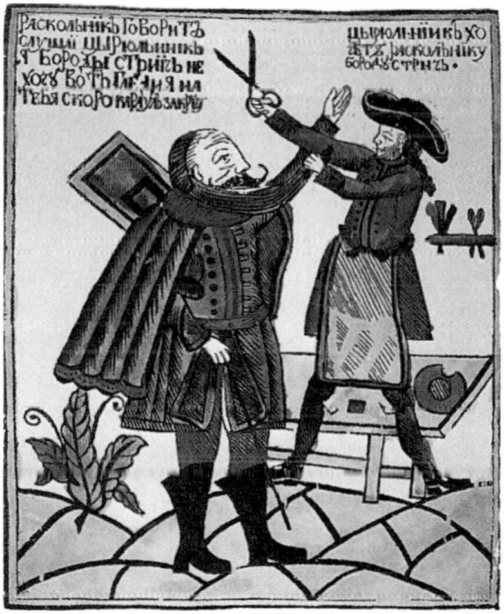
РАСКОЛЬНИКЪ ГОВОРИТЪ
СЛУШАЙ ЦЫРЮЛЬНИКЪ
Я БОРОДЫ СТРИЧЬ НЕ
ЦЫРЮЛЬНИКЪ ХО
БОРОДУ СТРИЧЬ

Above: In addition to taxes on the right to marry and wear a beard, Peter taxed mills, hats, cellars, and coffins.

Tax collectors, armed with scissors, were stationed at the gates of every city and throughout the rural provinces to crop the beards and mustaches of those who refused to pay the tax. Defiant wearers of illegal facial hair were sentenced to hard labor. Peter the Great and his successors carried on the taxing and cutting of Russians' beards until 1765, when Catherine the Great repealed the law.

Benjamin Franklin

A century later, Benjamin Franklin counted among his blessings that he could "set [his] own razor and shave [himself] perfectly well." Franklin disliked barbers just as much as he disliked beards.

"Human felicity," he wrote, "is produced not so much by great pieces of good fortune that seldom happen as by little advantages that occur every day. Thus, if you teach a poor young man to shave himself and keep his razor in order, you may contribute more to the happiness of his life than in giving him a thousand guineas. The money may be soon spent, the regret only remaining of having foolishly consumed it; but in the other case, he escapes the frequent vexation of waiting for barbers and of their sometimes dirty fingers, offensive breaths and dull razors; he shaves when most convenient to him and enjoys daily the pleasure of its being done with a good instrument."

Beau Brummell

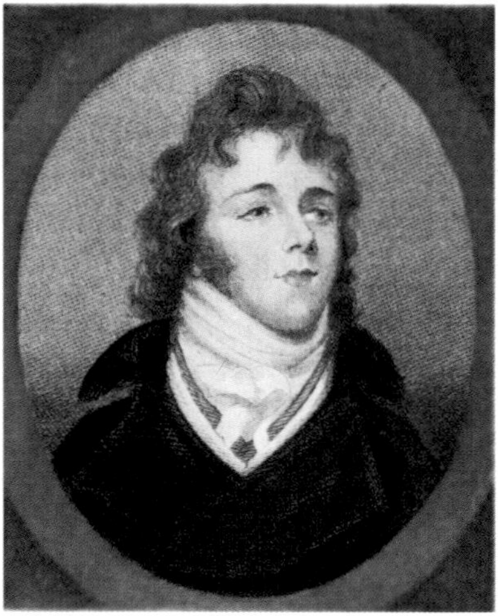

George Bryan "Beau" Brummell (1778–1840) was born without land or fortune. Nevertheless, he became the friend of the Prince Regent, later George IV, and was himself the acknowledged emperor of English dandyism. Known for his impeccable grooming, his elegant manners and style of dress, Brummell was reputed to shave his face several times a day and pluck out errant hairs with tweezers. He had the same high standards for his head as for his face. Reputed to employ three separate coiffeurs, one to do his front locks, a second his side locks, and a third to take care of the hair at the back of his head, he wielded personal style like a weapon. Brummell died in poverty in a French madhouse. At least one straight razor and one safety razor blade have borne his name.

ARTHUR SCHOPENHAUER

Arthur Schopenhauer (1788–1860), the German philosopher who

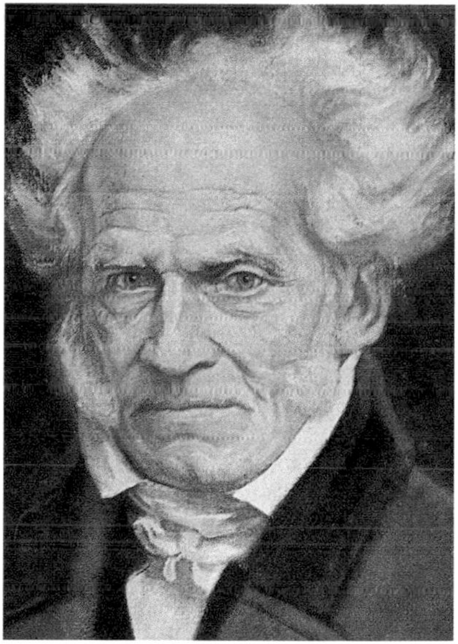

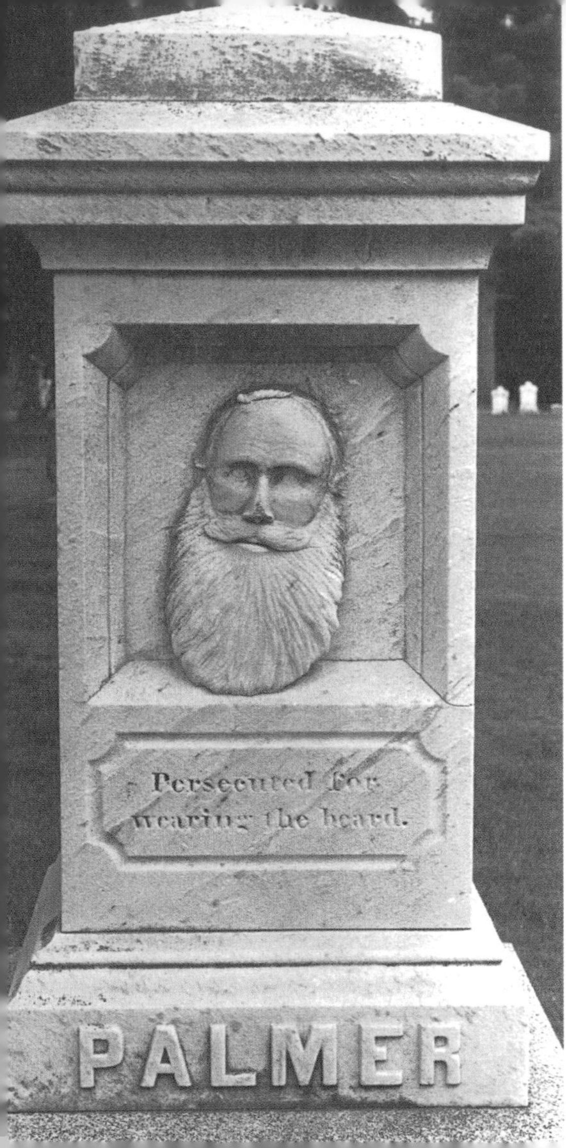

believed the world as we perceive it to be a malignant illusion that seduces us into wrongly perpetuating life, preached the ascetic and chaste life. He was also a vociferous advocate of shaving. "Just look at the profile of a bearded man while he eats," he wrote. All men should be clean-shaven. Beards masked the face and protected the criminal. Ideally, they would be forbidden by law.

JOSEPH PALMER

Born in Massachusetts in 1789, Joseph Palmer fought in the War of 1812, took up farming, and for reasons best known to himself, grew a beard in 1830. His farm was a success. His beard was not. Small boys threw stones to make this clear. The pastor of his church scolded him, chastising his beard as a satanic device.

After ten years of finding Palmer's beard intolerable, men armed with shears, brush, soap, and razor fell upon him. Palmer fought them off and was fined for "unprovoked assault," but he declined to pay and was jailed. Eventually his plight became known throughout the state and a movement to have him released was successful. His tombstone records history's verdict.

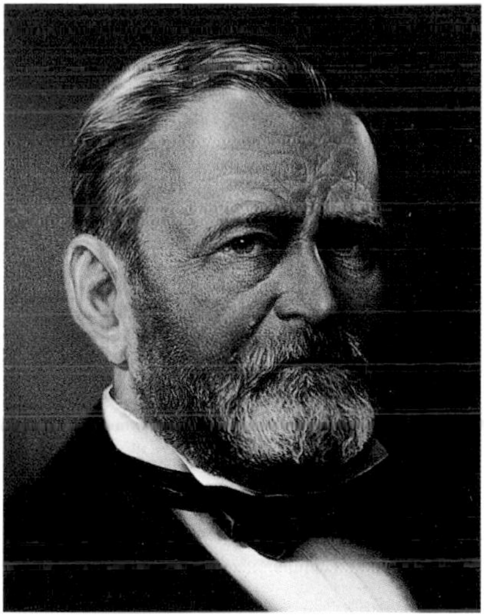

Above: Former President Ulysses S. Grant

U.S. Presidents

European kings set the style for beards and beardlessness. American presidents followed the fashion of their time. In the first half of the nineteenth century, being clean-shaven was the norm for Americans. Uncle Sam himself didn't grow chin whiskers until 1858, just before the national style changed. Abraham Lincoln grew his own beard two years later at the age of fifty-two, and except for his immediate successor, Andrew Johnson,

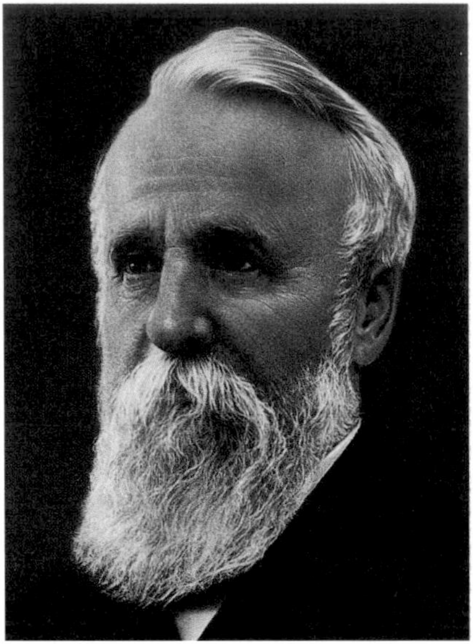

Above: President with the longest beard, Rutherford B. Hayes

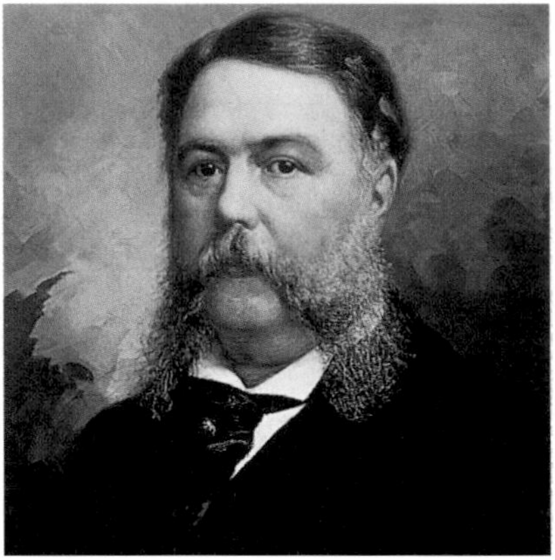

Above: President with the bushiest facial hair, Chester A. Arthur

there wasn't a clean-shaven president for thirty years.

Ulysses S. Grant had a neat beard himself and the hairiest cabinet in history. Rutherford B. Hayes had the longest beard of any president, while Chester A. Arthur's side-whiskers and mustache would have taken first prize for bushiness. Grover Cleveland came to the White House with a mustache, was defeated by the last of the bearded presidents, Benjamin Harrison, then returned for a second term with his mustache intact. By this time, the public health movement was gaining in strength, and men

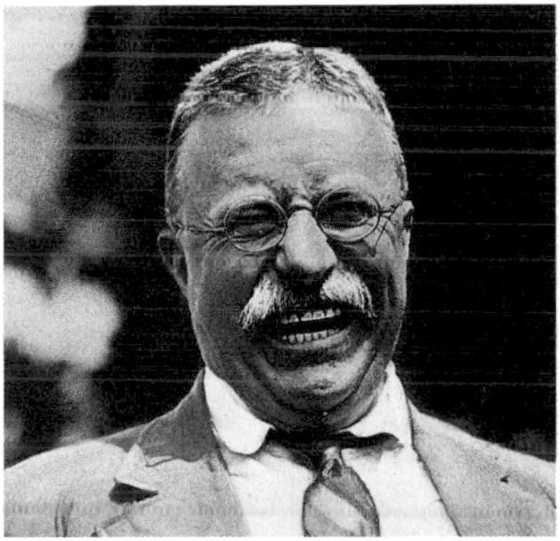

were entreated to shave their beards so as not to bring germs into the home. William McKinley shaved; Theodore Roosevelt and William Howard Taft had mustaches; since then, the White House has known only clean cheeks and upper lips.

Left: Theodore Roosevelt
Below: Franklin D. Roosevelt

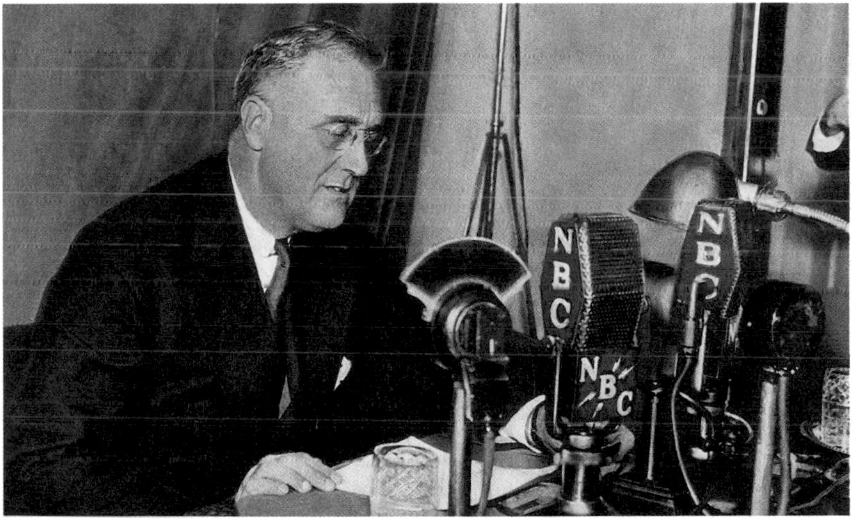

ABRAHAM LINCOLN

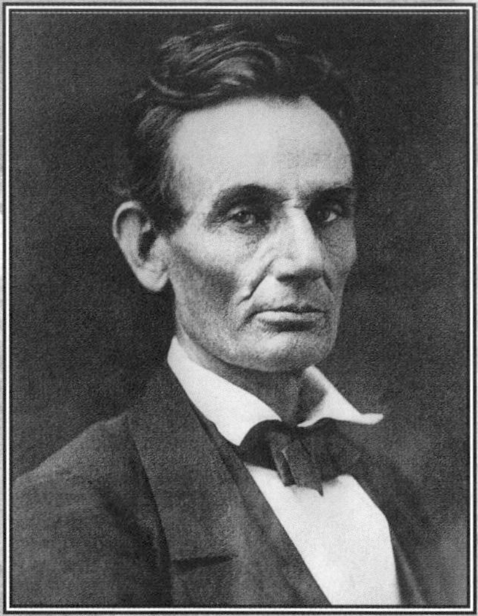

In October 1860, Abraham Lincoln received the following letter from little Grace Bedell on how to get more votes for the presidency by growing a beard:

"Dear Sir My father has just [come] home from the fair and brought home your picture. I am a little girl only eleven years old, but want you should be President of the United States very much so I hope you won't think me very bold to write to such a great man as you are. Have you any little girls about as large as I am if so give them my love and tell her to write to me if you cannot answer this letter. I have got 4 brothers and part of them will vote for you any way and if you will let your whiskers grow I will try and get the rest of them to vote for you and then you would be President. . . . I think that rail fence around your picture makes it look very pretty. I have got a little baby sister she is nine weeks old and is just as cunning as can be. . . ."

Lincoln replied, "My dear little Miss. Your very agreeable letter of the 15th is received. I regret the necessity of saying I have no daughters. I have three sons—one seventeen, one nine, and one seven, years of age. They, with their mother, constitute my whole family.

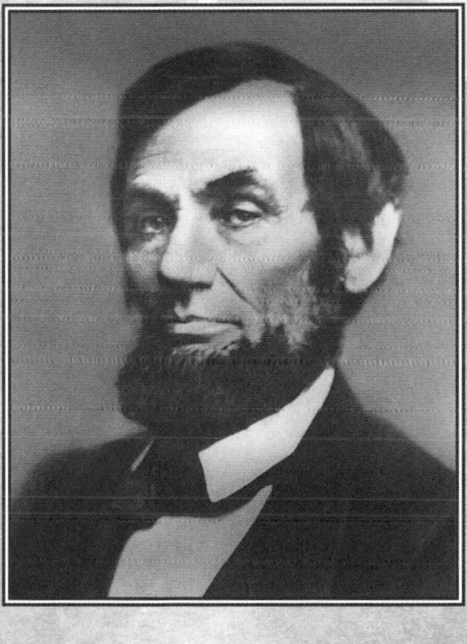

As to the whiskers, never having worn any, do you not think people would call it a piece of silly affect[at]ion if I were to begin it now? Your very sincere well-wisher etc."

Two months later, traveling by train to his inauguration in Washington, Lincoln visited Westfield, New York, where the Bedell family lived. Proud bearer of a new beard, he addressed the people who had come to greet him and acknowledged the girl's part in his decision to let his whiskers grow so as to improve his appearance. Was she in the crowd? He should like to see her. A boy pointed her out. "Amid yells of delight from the excited crowd" Lincoln planted "several hearty kisses" on Grace's cheek.

Benito Mussolini

In 1926, Benito Mussolini's (1883–1945) political ambitions had yet to be realized, but he was already a dedicated Gillette user. He told the United Press Association: I have "to use a new blade every time I shave, for there are no blades made that can stand more than one shave on my beard." But he had political reasons for shaving every day as well. "I am anti-whiskers. Fascism is anti-whiskers. Whiskers are a sign of decadence. Glance at the busts of the great Roman Emperors and you will find them all clean-shaven—Caesar, Augustus. When the decline of Roman glory began, whiskers came into style. It is true of all periods. The Renaissance was a beardless period. Whiskers were the rule in the old decadent regime, which Fascism replaces with youth of clean-shaven faces."

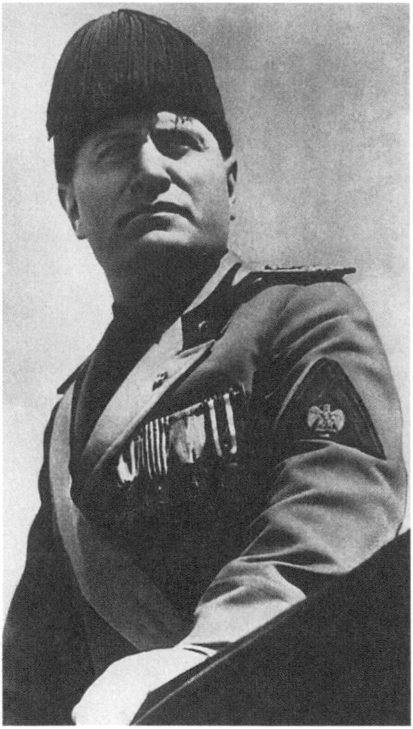

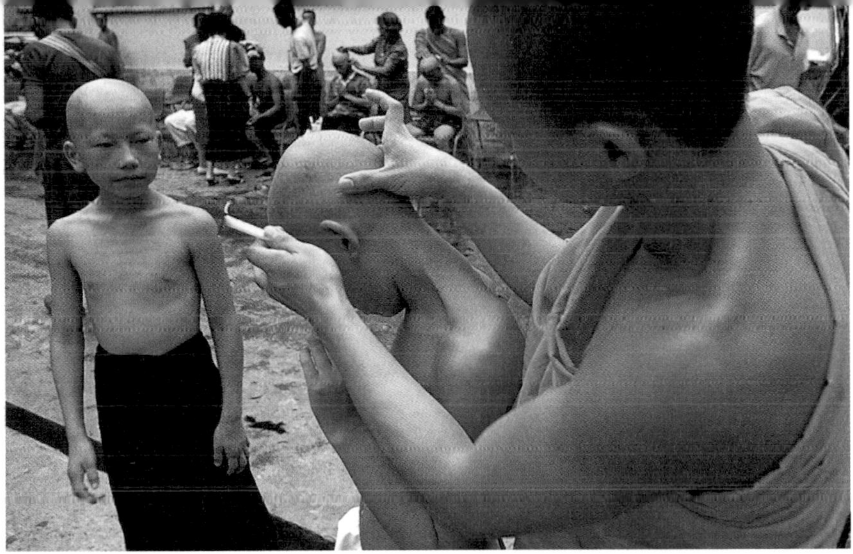

Above: For young Thai monks, head shaving represents a renunciation of worldly attachments.

Divine Sanction

Faith trumps fashion. Sometimes an individual can influence the way other men tend their chins by his example—Beau Brummell—or by his power—Peter the Great. Usually it takes an entire society to decide what it wants beards or beardlessness to signify. Every so often, however, more is required. Special situations—collective identity, mourning, battle—require special rules. And to make these rules stick, they're usually given a divine sanction and are couched in solemn tones.

Muslims and Beards

Islam does not speak with a single monolithic voice about beards and shaving. The most pious Muslim men will let their beards grow because, according to Islamic teaching, it is in keeping with man's nature.

Allah's messenger, Muhammad, instructed his first followers to cut their mustaches and let their beards grow in order to distinguish themselves from the long-mustached Magians, fire-worshipers from Persia. To Muslims, the beard is also a major distinction between men and women. Men who shave their beards are imitating women. Worse yet are the men who shave their beards to please their wives, evidence of how far the world has come from the pure state in which Allah created it.

The most conservative Muslims believe that shaving the beard constitutes a kind of impermissible self-mutilation. However, there are occasions in Islamic life when all men must shave. During the hajj before passing into the sacred territory of Mecca, a pilgrim must be in a state of ritual purity. For a man, this involves trim-

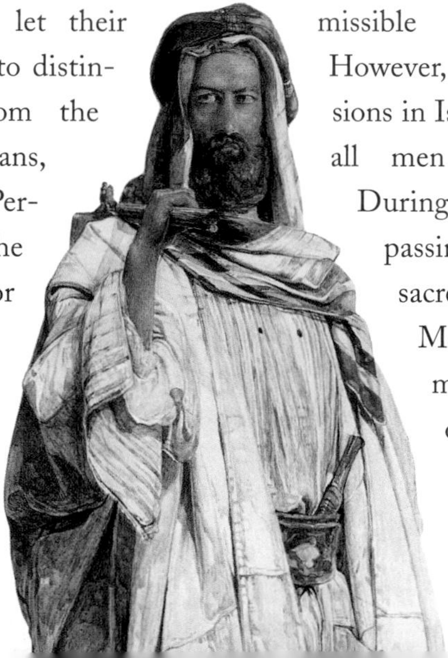

Right: Painting by artist Carl Friedrich Heinrich Werner (1808–94)

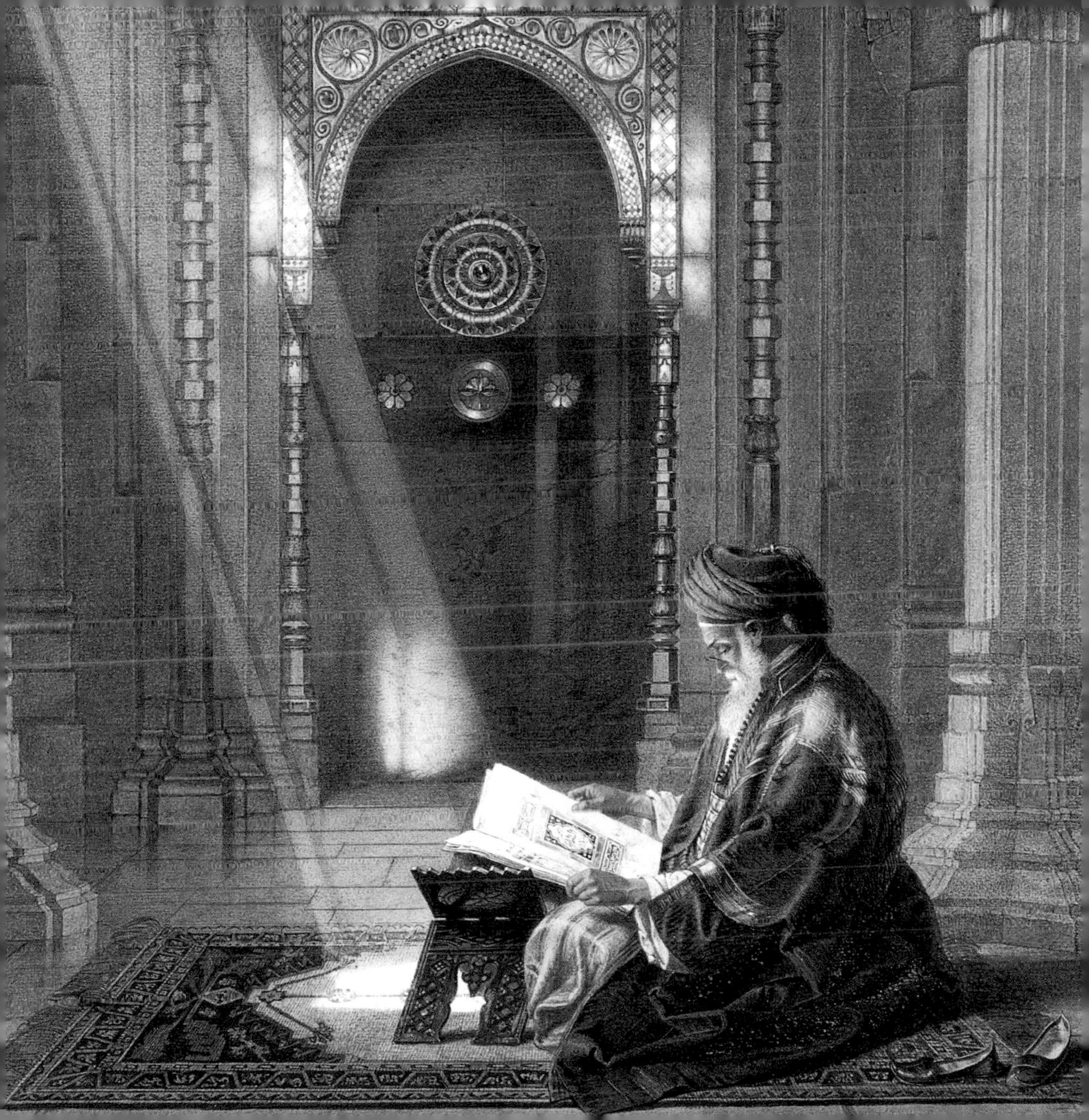

ming the fingernails, shaving off beard and mustache, and removing all bodily hair. While in this state of purity (*iḥrām*), the pilgrim is forbidden to use perfumes or carry symbols of personal wealth. Until the pilgrimage has been completed, hair and nails may not be cut again.

Sitting Shiva

Going unshaven for the observant Jew is a part of mourning. When a family member has died, the immediate family sits shiva for seven days. Mourners sit on low stools or the floor instead of chairs, cover all mirrors, and abstain from wearing leather shoes. They avoid worldly activities—people mustn't shave or cut their hair—and they do nothing for comfort or pleasure, such as bathe, have sex, put on fresh clothing, or study Torah that is unrelated to mourning and grief.

Leviticus 19:27, "Ye shall not round the corners of your heads, neither shalt thou mar the corners of thy beard" is a significant text for Orthodox Jews and Hassidim. "Marring" is understood to mean "shaving with a razor"; using scissors or electric shavers that imitate the action of scissors is acceptable.

There is an absolute prohibition on cutting the hair that grows at the temple and upper sideburns, the *peyos.* It can be trimmed, it just can't be cut off entirely.

Amish Beards

A Dutch Mennonite who observed the Amish in the early 1700s said of them: "They are a sturdy folk by nature, able to endure great hardships, with long, untrimmed beards, simple clothes, heavy shoes. . . . They are very zealous in serving God . . . and are very sincere in all they do."

Nearly three hundred years later, their spade beards, along with the old-fashioned clothing and the horse-drawn wagons, are the outward expressions of a faith that rejects worldliness. When Catholics were warring with Protestants and Protestants were warring with each other, the Amish were persecuted for their belief that true faith involved a literal reading of the Bible and for preaching that reading to the interested and the uninterested alike. Such literal-mindedness was not well received by either Catholics or other Protestants in post-Reformation Europe. Their early enthusiasm dimmed in the face of imprisonment and execution and in reaction the Amish withdrew from the world, first farming small holdings in the mountains of Switzerland and southern Germany, later sending groups to settle in Pennsylvania and Ohio.

The Sikhs

Like the Amish, the way Sikh men in India wear their hair and beards symbolizes their membership in the community of faith. Followers of the guru Gobind Singh (1666–1708) formed the Khalsa (the pure) and adopted five badges of membership, known as the five K's: *kes,* wearing the hair long and keeping the beard unshorn; *kangha,* the comb required to keep the hair, typically covered by a turban, tidy;

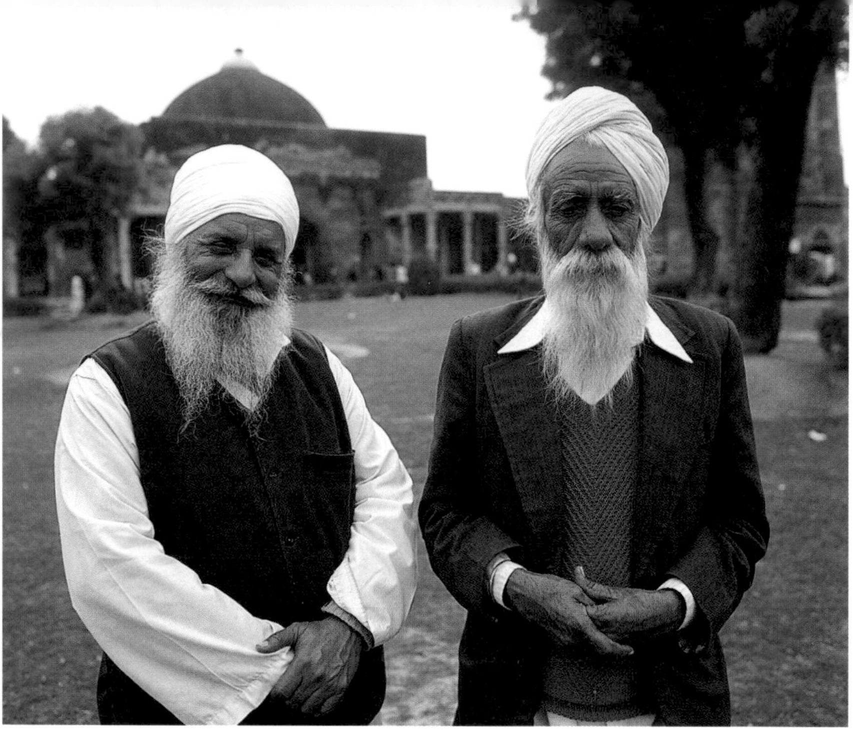

kach, knee-length breeches, as were worn by soldiers; *kara,* steel bracelets worn on the right wrist; and *kirpan,* a dagger.

Unshorn hair and untrimmed beards are still such an essential part of the Sikh identity that when Sikhs and Hindus were at odds in the Punjab State in the early 1980s, the greatest humiliation a mob could inflict on a captured Sikh was to cut off his hair and beard.

The U.S Marine Corps is like a religion with regard to the loyalty it inspires. And like a religion, it makes it easy for the faithful to know what they must do. According to written rules:

"No male Marine will be required to have his hair clipped to the scalp except while he is undergoing recruit training or when such action is prescribed by a medical officer. This does not prohibit a male Marine from having his hair clipped to the scalp if he so desires.

"The face will be clean-shaven, except that a mustache may be worn. When worn, the mustache will be neatly trimmed . . . and the individual length of a mustache hair fully extended must not exceed ½ inch.

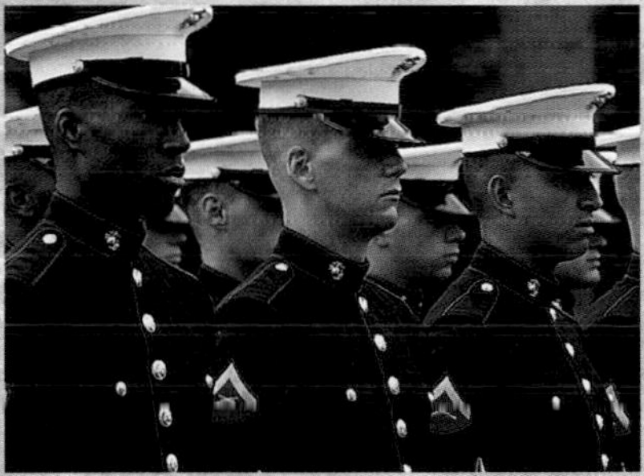

"Except for a mustache, eyebrows, and eyelashes, hair may be grown on the face only when a medical officer has determined that shaving is temporarily harmful to the individual's health."

"No male Marine will be required to have his chest hair clipped except that which is so long as to protrude in an unsightly manner above the collar of the long sleeve khaki shirt."

A man who lives to be eighty will spend some 2,965 hours of his life—about four months—shaving. By the time he's been at it for a couple of years, he barely has to think about what he's doing. He could shave in his sleep and, some mornings, he does. So what goes through his mind as he shears off the night's production of whiskers? Lord Byron, we're told, composed poetry while he was being shaved. How about the guy shaving at the gym? What's going on behind his furrowed brow? Or your twin brother? Are his thoughts the same as yours? What *do* men think about while they shave? A random sampling of seasoned shavers yielded the following answers.

The Professor

Except for touch-up, most of my shaving is done in the shower. There I have some of my best thoughts about science and the world, organize lectures, think about the day's laboratory work, compose doggerel, and generally *get going.*

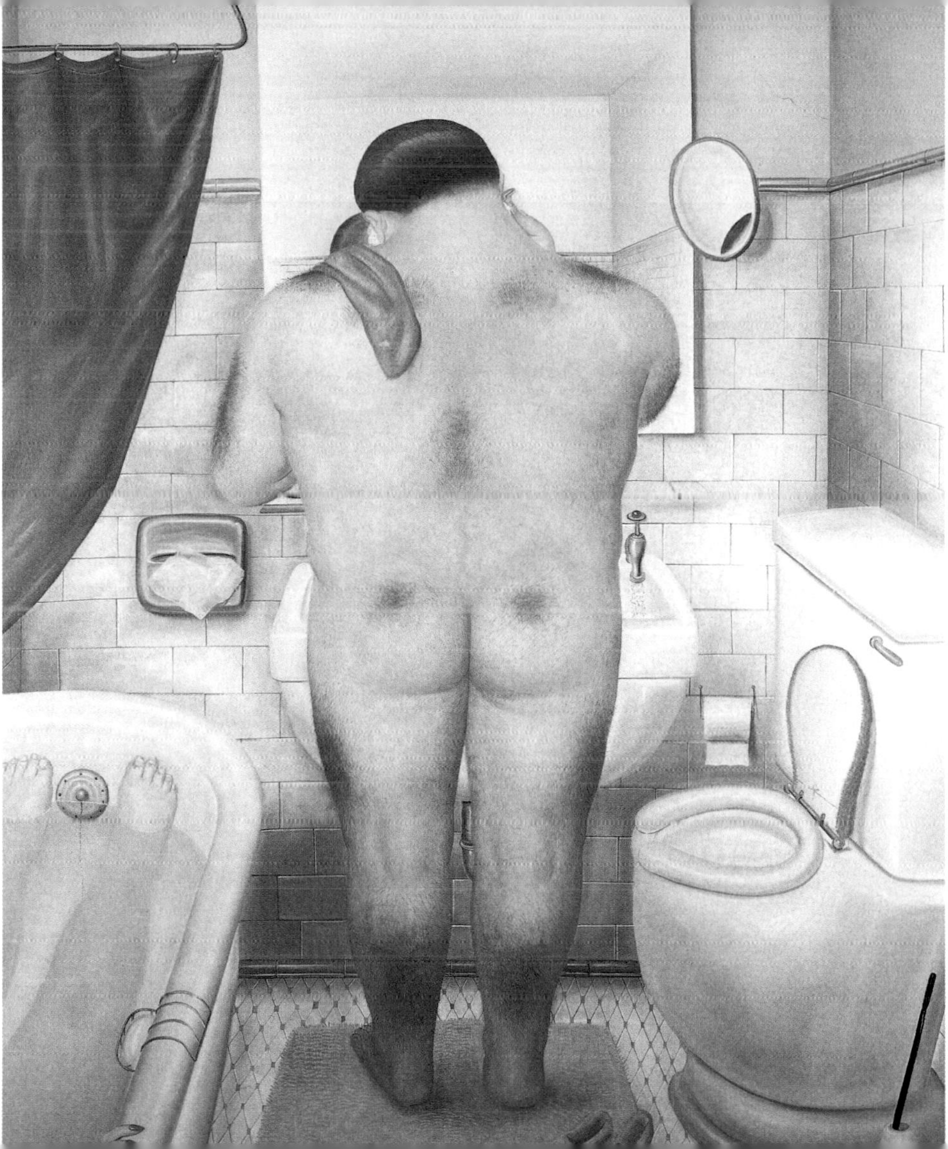

The Conflicted Pessimist

First and foremost, I shave only when absolutely required and generally hate it. If I would look other than like a homeless person with some sort of horrid skin disease, I would grow a beard. But alas, due to facial scars inflicted by various male rites of passage (e.g., taking it on the chin with a hockey stick), there are large areas that produce no hair at all.

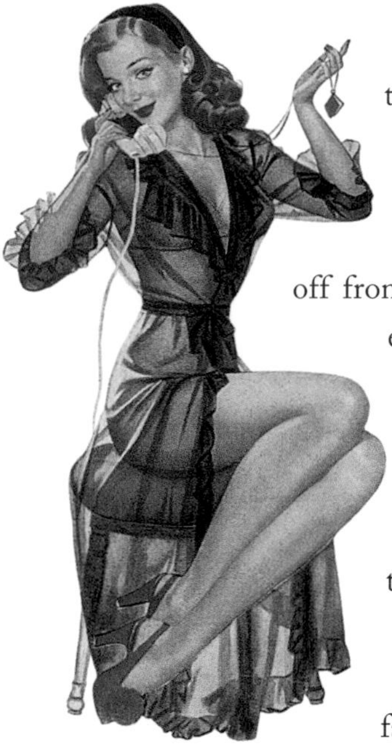

I found years ago that the shaving experience lent itself to deep neurotic musings about all the painful things that would likely befall me at work. So nowadays I use that time to fool myself into thinking I'm about to have a spectacular day, as the alternative had me whipped into a frenetic fit before I set off from the breakfast table each day. Strange, but highly effective. A product of the nineties, to be sure.

The Fastidious Dreamer

Sometimes I shave twice. I use an electric razor for ten minutes. Then, if I really want to feel clean-shaven, I get out the can of Barbasol and the razor and do it all over again. For some peculiar I-can't-fathom-why reason, certain romantic liaisons of the past seem to come back to me as I'm staring into the mirror. As I'm doing the upstroke against my cheek, say, I'll think of Madame X or Y. Not of sex, actually, just of the person. Perhaps, like acupuncture on the foot, there are certain sensitive nerves in the face that are hot-wired back to the brain's memory banks.

The Ecumenical Buddhist

I start mumbling Tibetan mantras as I wet my face with warm water. While I briefly lather with soap, I recite a favorite short sutra and take a momentary look heavenward to ask for blessings from both Siva and Allah. During the actual shaving I hold my breath with one strong powerful exhalation at the end of the process. As I wash the razor I give thanks to the fact that I already look younger than I did when I awoke.

The Diplomat

This is my most productive time, the moment I remember the most important thing I must do during the day ahead. Like, sign a contract, or clip my nails, or plan my jogging schedule for the weekend, or remember to send a poisonous memo to some evil colleague. Often the wording of that memo will come clear to me only through the haze of the moist bathroom air, bringing into focus the really important things like hygiene for myself and poison for others.

The Average Joe

I don't do anything while I shave besides let my mind wander over the various trivial details that seem to fill our heads most of the time—how are the Red Sox doing? Is this blade getting dull already? Do I need to iron a shirt? etc.

The Bleeder

I sometimes look into the mirror, observe evidence of aging (God, I'm really not twenty-five anymore!), and wonder how I arrived at forty, improperly trained in the subtle art of face scraping, and life in general, by my father or anyone else. Self-improvement? Inasmuch as I am stimulating white blood cell production by cutting myself, thereby boosting my immune system function, yes. On a good day it is a meditative interlude without excessive blood loss.

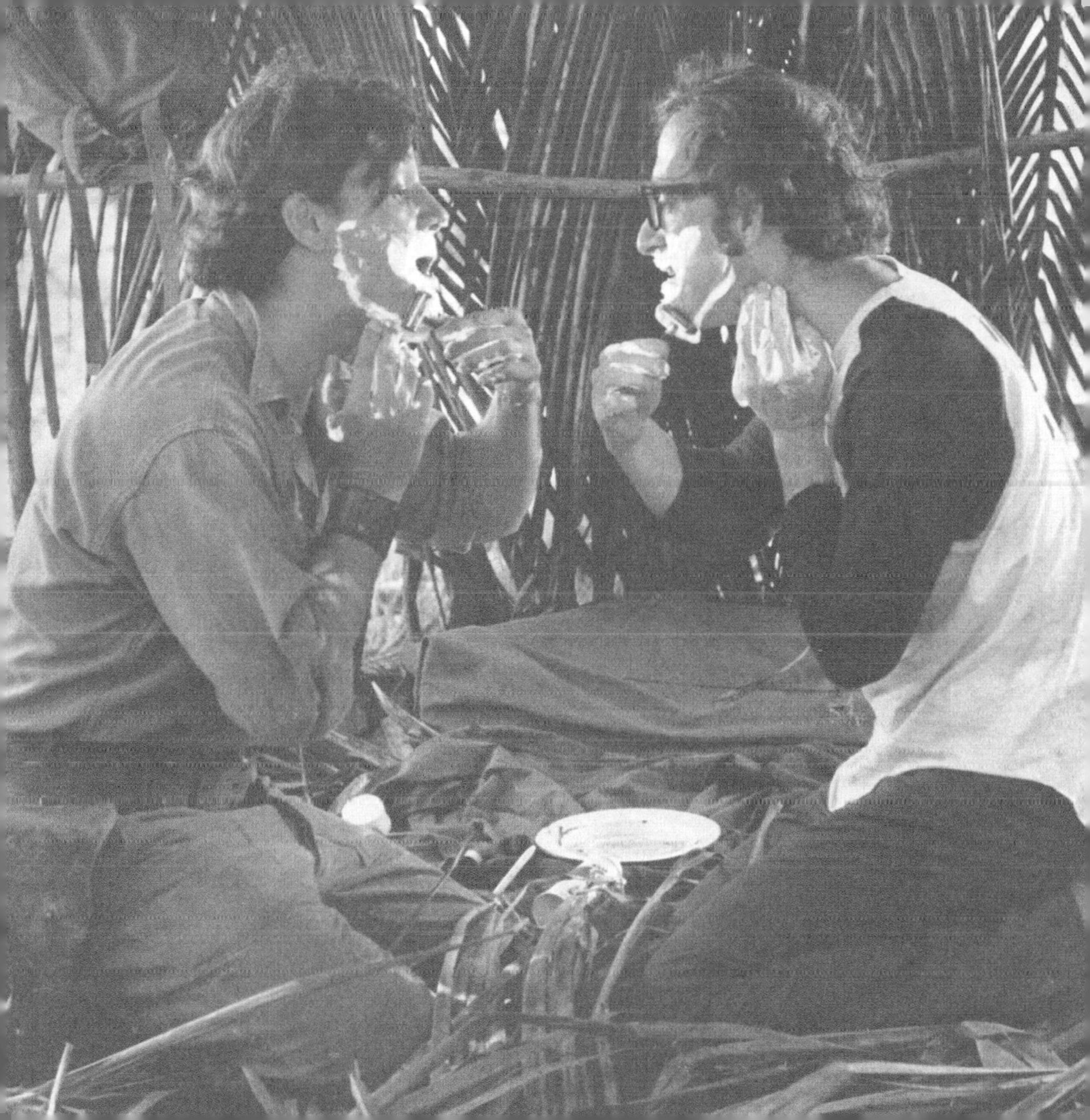

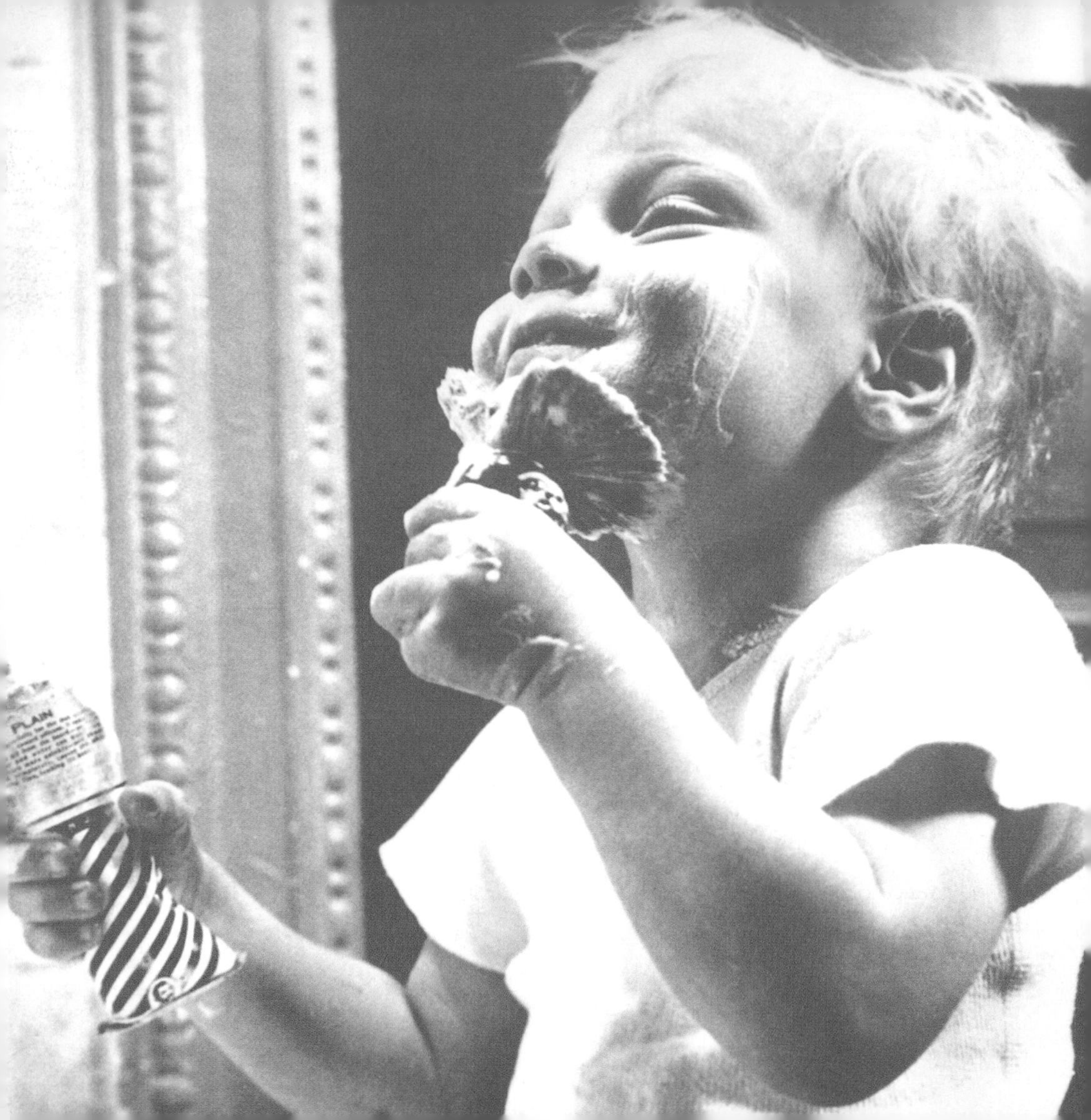
PLAIN

HOW TO SHAVE YOUR FACE

Indeed, when one considers what variety of sounds can be uttered by the windpipe, in the compass of a very small aperture, we may be convinced how many degrees of difference there may be in the application of the razor.

James Boswell, *Life of Samuel Johnson*

Every man shaves himself in a different fashion. And although individual techniques vary, shavers have a common goal that, like the incest taboo and the prevalence of gravity, is practically a cultural universal: a clean shave, a close shave, a shave that doesn't cause suffering while it's being performed or shame and humiliation when it's finished. Mood, temperament, and occasion may influence the way a man shaves on a given day but the basic principles of a good shave are plain and simple.

Left: A good technique and a good attitude, acquired young, will give a man a good shave at any age.

The Perfect Wet Shave

1. Soften your beard with water. Go for a swim. Stand in the shower for five minutes. Soak a washcloth in warm water and apply it to your face, go do something else, then come back and repeat the procedure. The point is to give your whiskers time to get wet enough to swell up a bit; they'll shear off more easily, and your razor blade will last longer.

If you have a tough beard or sensitive skin, standing in the shower is a particularly good idea. It's a perfect place to shave, especially if you have a nonfogging mirror in there with you.

2. If your beard is really soft and your blade really sharp, you can shave with hot water alone. Applying shaving foam or gel or cream keeps the beard wet and makes it easier for the razor to glide over the surface of your skin without cutting it. So does plain old soap, albeit less effectively.

3. The received wisdom is that long, smooth strokes produce better results than short, jerky ones, and that shaving with the lie of the beard produces better results than shaving against it. Every man has to find the method that suits him best; however, some basics do apply. You want to rinse the razor regularly so the blade doesn't clog with soap and stubble, and you should put in a new blade once the

one you've been using for a week or ten days starts to drag.

Ideally, you should go over each area a single time, but the odds are good that you will have missed a patch here or there. Unless your skin is broken out or chronically sensitive, it won't hurt to make a second pass over these patches at a different, crosswise angle. Most beards are toughest on the upper lip and the chin, so leave these for last.

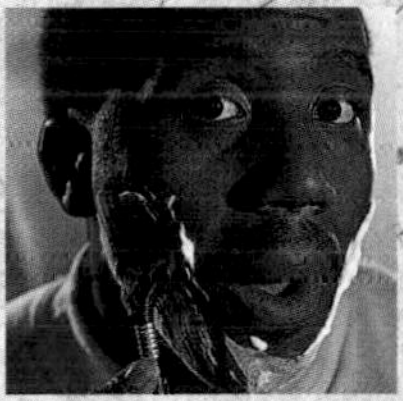

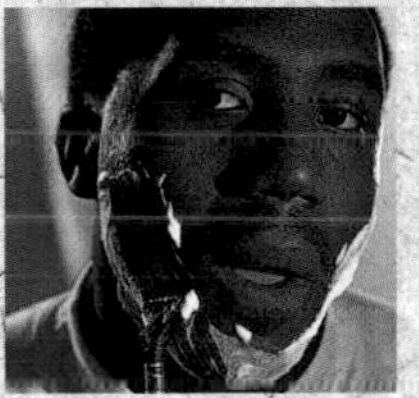

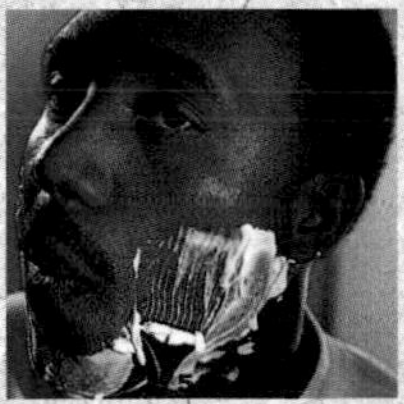

4. Once you're satisfied with the shave, rinse with cold water, pat your face dry, and apply some kind of aftershave product. The choice is up to you but the same skin care experts who caution against shaving with painfully hot water or shaving too closely say that you shouldn't be putting alcohol on your skin. You aren't doing your face any favors if it's stinging. After all, you've just shaved off a thin slice of epidermis and an aftershave that burns is nature's way of letting you know the slice wasn't thin enough. Having just scraped your skin, you now want to soothe it, not slap it.

For Contrarians

The shaving method patented in 1942 by New York inventor Peter N. Peters may be of interest to those of you who want to break all the rules. Mr. Peters recommended washing, lathering, and rinsing the face with cold water, but shaving with a hot blade—as hot as bearable. Rather than making long clean strokes with the razor, he suggested making sharp rapid ones. The reasoning behind the invention is that hot water and lathering make the skin flabby and render the hair so limp it cannot be properly sheared off by the razor.

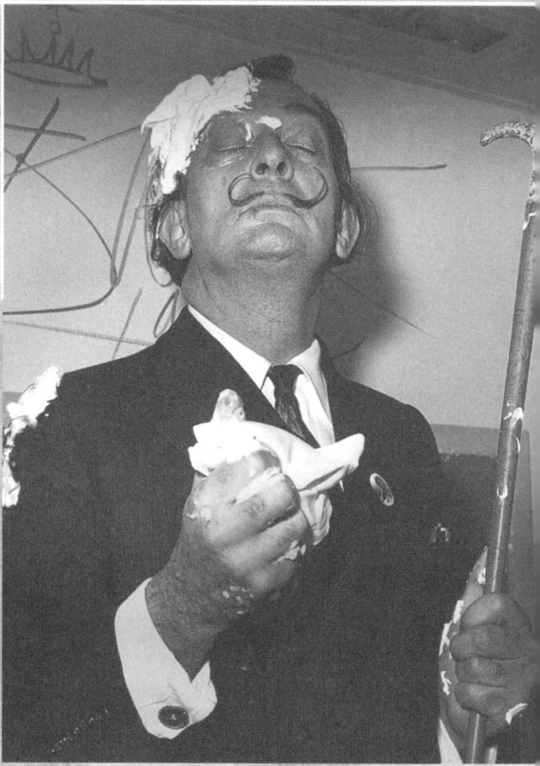

Shaving with an Electric Shaver

Electric shavers have either a rotary head—circular cutters that rotate behind round combs—or a foil head blades that move back and forth and are covered by one or more flexible metal foils. You move a foil shaver up and down your face, a rotary shaver in a circular motion. Foil heads have to be replaced fairly often; a rotary head may last for years. Either type can have adjustable settings so you can regulate the closeness of the shave.

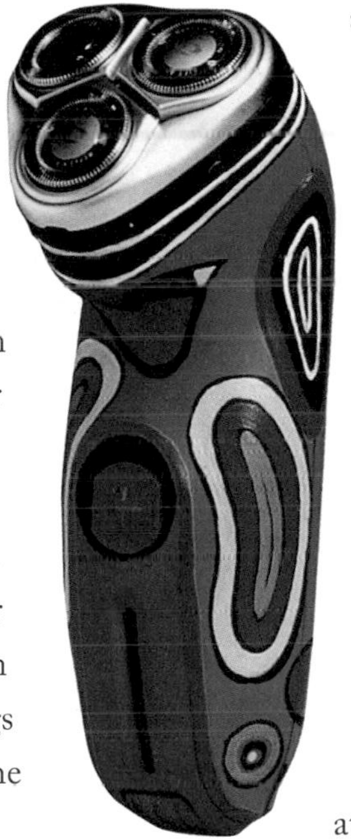

Shaving with an electric shaver has its merits. Your face stays dry, you can shave pretty much anywhere you like, and unless you're a borderline obsessive and go over your face again and again and again, you can't even get razor burn.

The drawbacks? Electric shavers cost more, and no matter what you read or see on television, men with tough beards will never get as close a shave with an electric shaver as with a wet razor. Some tips:

Shave against the lie of your beard and don't press down hard. If the shaver you're using generates a little heat and you have sensitive skin, shave the tenderest areas first before the shaver heats up.

If your skin is oily, use a pre-shave preparation that will dry up surface moisture and ready your

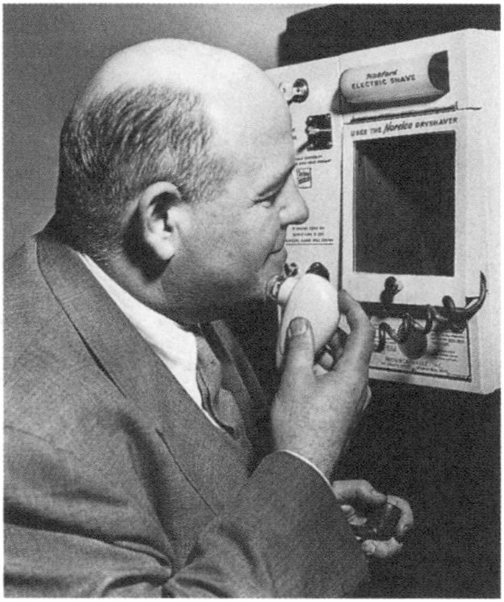

Above: In 1950, coin-operated electric shavers made it convenient for the man on the move to take care of his five o'clock shadow.

whiskers to be mowed down. A dry and therefore brittle hair is more susceptible than a wet one to the shearing action of an electric shaver.

Keep your shaver clean. On foil shavers, you can usually lift off the head frame that holds the screen and brush the whisker dust from the underside. Below the screen is the cutter and this part has to be brushed off with the manufacturer's cleaning brush.

With a rotary shaver, same drill. Once a week (or more often if necessary), brush whiskers from the comb slots. Then lift off the razor head assembly and brush hair from the underside of the three cutters and the razor chamber. Don't rap the heads on the sink to get whiskers out or you may damage the instrument.

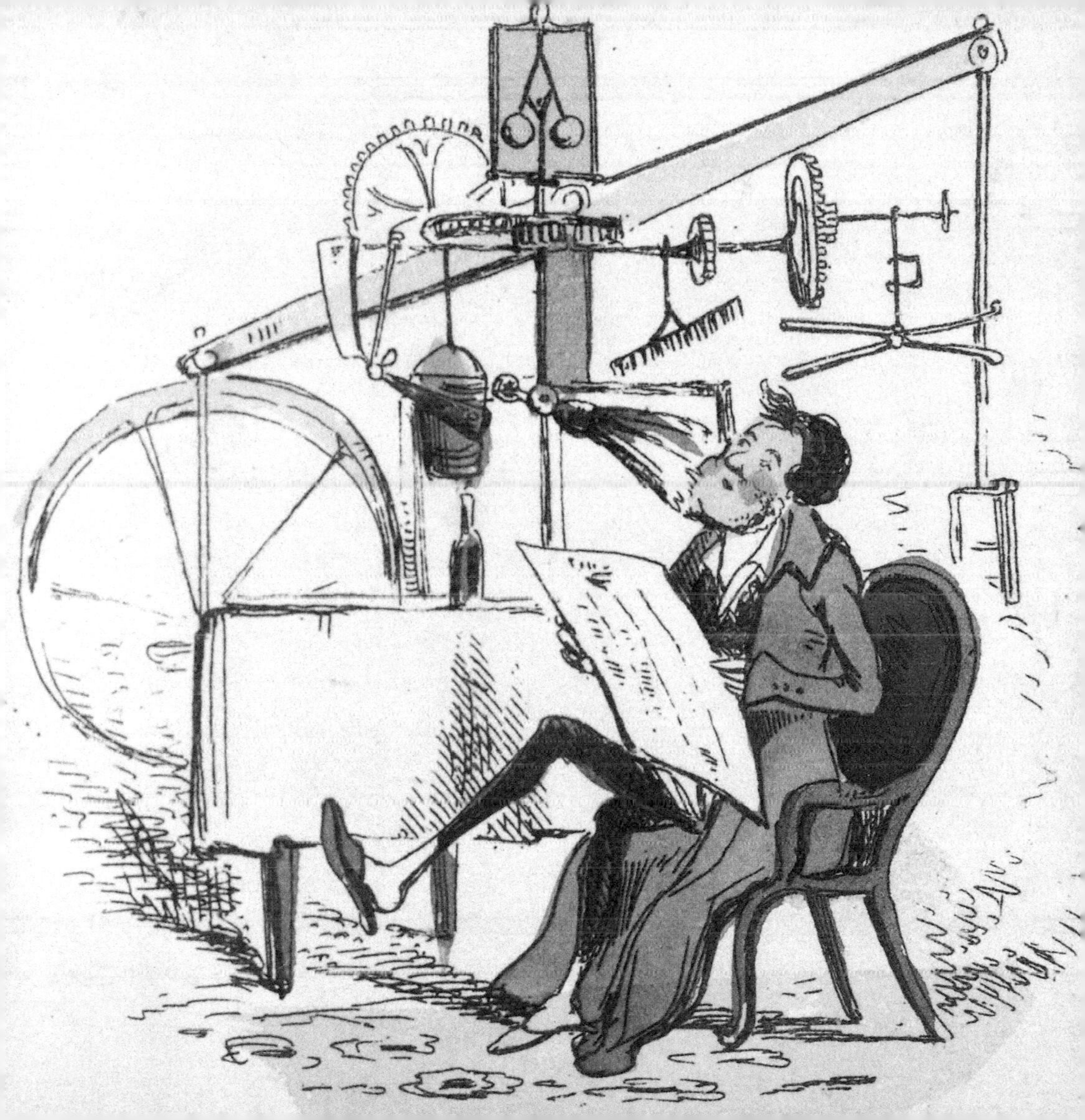

If you're switching from one brand of shaver to another or from wet to dry, give your face time to adjust. It may take two or three weeks before you get the most your electric shaver has to offer.

Further Dos and Don'ts

If you have sensitive skin, try an electric shaver first to get rid of the major stubble, then go back with a wet razor and a light touch to get the closer shave an electric shaver doesn't give. Since it's partly the drag of the razor across the skin that's irritating, make as few passes as possible. Over the weekend, give your face a rest from shaving; that would be beneficial too.

If your skin has a tendency to break out or you nick easily, choose an alcohol-free, unscented after-shave balm. And using a moisturizer at night will make shaving easier the next morning.

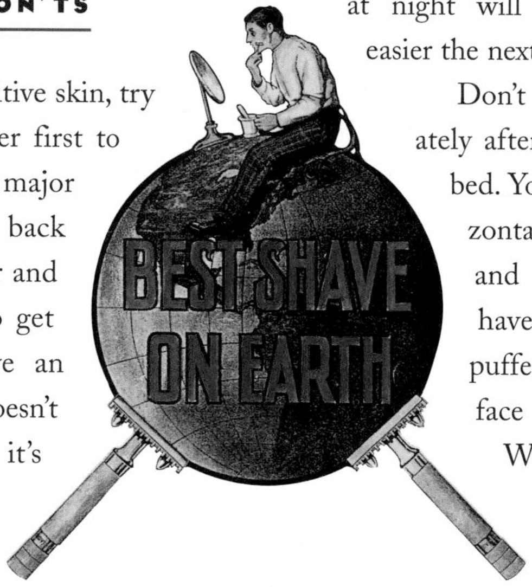

Don't shave immediately after rolling out of bed. You've been horizontal all night long, and body fluids have pooled and puffed up the surface of your skin. Wait awhile until this puffiness dissipates.

A man who maintains a three-day growth of stubble for weeks and months on end does not achieve that look with an electric razor. He uses electric clippers set on their lowest setting. Stubble works on a man's face the way contouring makeup works on a woman's, creating shadows and definition absent from his clean-shaven visage.

Stubble makes you look as if you just got out of bed, which can be read as (1) kinda sexy or (2) kinda disoriented. Whichever message you wish to send, don't contradict it with overly neat edges. Stubble's message is I'm hipper than most and I've got better things to do than shave. So do them and leave those edges alone.

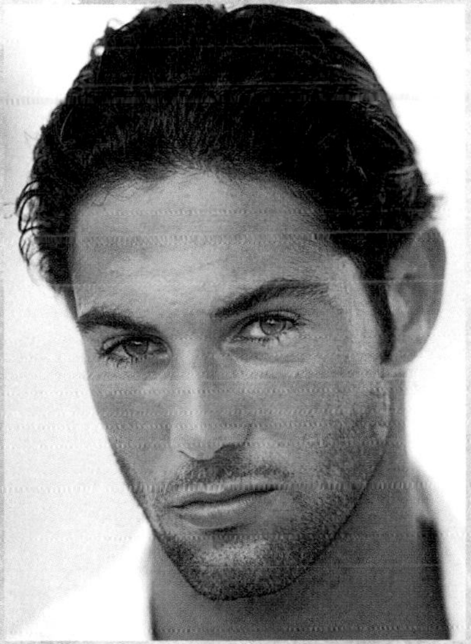

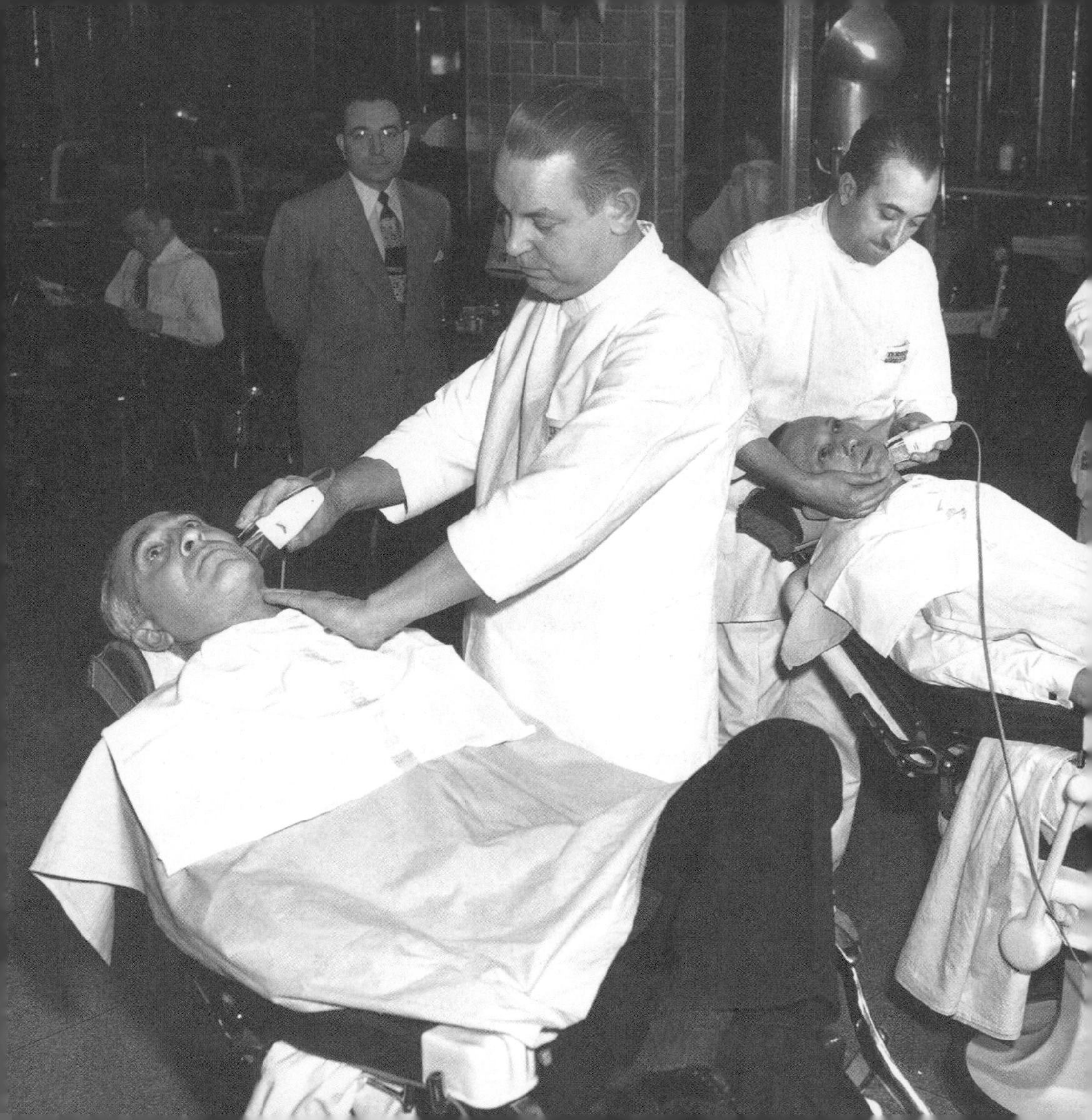

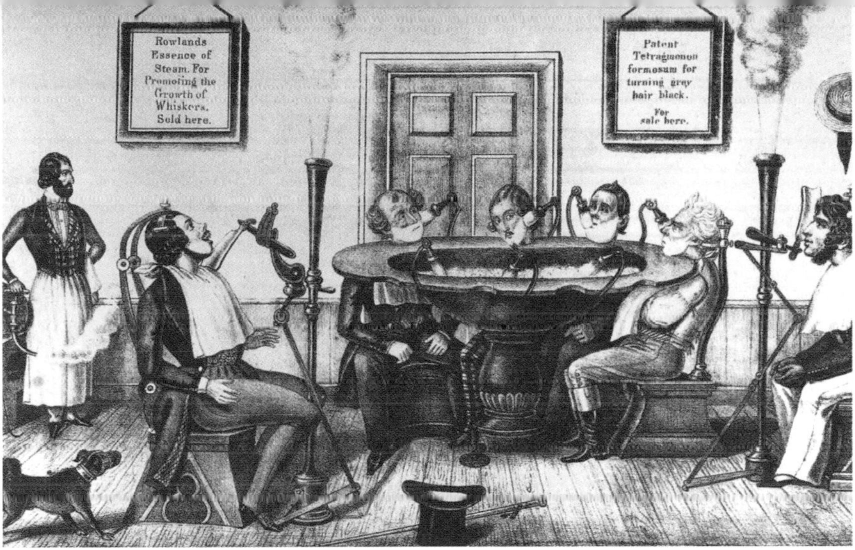
Rowlands Essence of Steam. For Promoting the Growth of Whiskers. Sold here.
Patent Tetragmenon formosum for turning grey hair black. For sale here.

Left: In the dry summer of 1949, New York City asked its citizens to forgo baths and wet shaves on Fridays. Barbers cooperated. Above: Midway through the Industrial Revolution, a cartoonist concocts a "steam shaving shop" where barbers are replaced by shaving machines.

In an ideal world, we'd shave in the evening when the face is oilier and its owner is less rushed.

In general, you want to shave when your skin is least likely to suffer from irritation. Shave in the evening in the summer. Sunscreen may irritate freshly shaven skin, so may chlorine from the pool or salt from the ocean. Don't shave just before you work out; perspiration is highly alkaline and can make dry skin drier. Besides, you'll get a better shave after the post-workout shower.

If any mention of skin care

causes your testosterone level to drop, for a little over a dollar you can pick up a bottle of witch hazel at the drug store. It's 14 percent alcohol, is pleasantly astringent, and is also good for mosquito bites.

Razor Bumps

Good preparation, a decent razor, and a modicum of attention to skin care will for most men result in a satisfactory shave. Men with coarse, curly beards are going to have a harder time of it. Sooner or later, they're likely to develop the annoying condition known as razor bumps (*Pseudofolliculitisbarbae* or PFB). The condition is particularly severe among African-American men and men of southern Mediterranean origin.

PFB results when the barbed tip of a newly shorn beard hair curls back on itself and penetrates the surface of the skin. The body treats the hair as a foreign body and infection sets in. The resulting bump or bumps get nicked with every pass of the razor, aggravating the condition.

There's no cure but there are remedies. One remedy is to grow a beard. If personal preference or professional considerations make that solution unfeasible, another is to use an electric razor specifically designed for the problem.

If a man predisposed to PFB still prefers a wet razor, here are some precautions he can take to avoid ingrown hairs in the first place:

• Use an exfoliant. Massage the beard area in small circular motions with either a clean, soft toothbrush or a facial scrub. This motion sets up beard hairs to be shaved, dislodges hairs starting to grow in the wrong direction, and gets rid of dead cells at the same time. Better yet, plan ahead. Use a moisturizer that contains AHA, a natural fruit acid that does the same thing as a facial scrub, just a bit less vigorously.

• Dip your razor in alcohol before you shave.

• Shave with the grain.

• If you've shaved over an ingrown hair and it's become infected, use an antibacterial agent like salicylic acid. Once the infection has cleared up, the hair should release itself. But stop shaving this patch until your skin has healed.

• Use a translucent shaving cream; it will allow you to see sensitive areas and avoid reinjury.

• If you don't have to be perfectly clean-shaven, don't lean on the blade so hard. Try leaving a little whisker. Or shave at night. Take your time and your face will have the whole night to recover from your ministrations.

• If shaving continues to be a problem, try using a depilatory. But be careful; some can irritate skin that's already raw.

• If none of this works, rethink a beard.

HOW TO GROW A BEARD

It's easier to bear a child once a year
than to shave every day.

Old Russian proverb

Is shaving an utter misery for you? Does the vision of your stubble in the mirror every morning start making you unhappy the night before? Perhaps it's not so much the stubble as the chin underneath that you don't like. Too strong, too weak, too dimpled, too plain—whatever it is, you want a change. Or perhaps you're just curious about how you'd look with a beard.

Then you begin to think about it. If you grew a beard, it might change the way people look at you. You haven't had one up until now and things are going all right. If you were to grow a beard, your baby goddaughter might be frightened. Your parents might criticize it. Your girlfriend or boyfriend or wife—or all three—might be repulsed. Well, maybe so and maybe not, but you won't know until you try. Besides, it's your head, it's your face, and you won't be the first man in history to test-drive a beard.

Unlike some other experiments

in self-discovery, a beard is not forever. The barbed-wire tattoo around your bicep that seemed like a good idea at twenty-three may lose its appeal a decade later. A beard changes your appearance and allows you to change your mind.

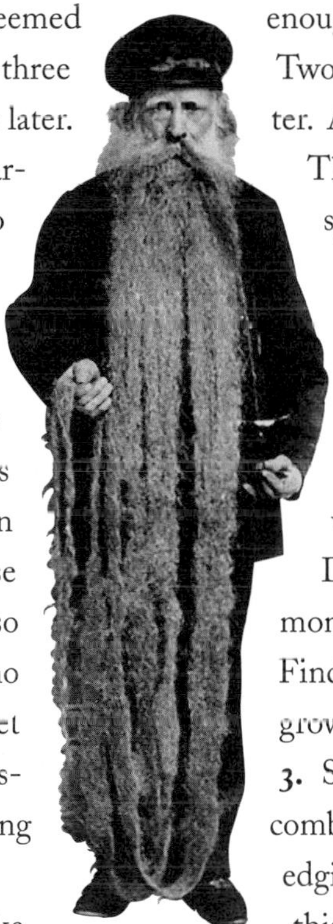

Sure, there are some poor excuses for beards out there—scary or pathetic or artificial-looking, beards that look less like a decision than like a long-term case of absentmindedness, not so much an afterthought as no thought at all. But don't let other people's mistakes discourage you from growing your own beard.

If you do decide to take the plunge, here are some things to keep in mind:

1. A weekend isn't quite long enough to start the process. Two weeks' vacation is better. A month is better yet. That way you'll be spared your co-workers' daily comments about its progress.

2. Patience is a virtue and you can cultivate that virtue with your new beard. Don't shave at all for a month. Don't even trim it. Find out what you can grow first.

3. Shaping a beard is like a combination of topiary and edging. Since you're new at this, have a barber help you define a "neck line," the point

where the beard stops and you start shaving, and advise you on how to shape all that new growth.

4. If it looks as if you might keep the beard around for a while, invest in clippers or an electric beard trimmer and follow the instructions. If you're frugal or undecided about the beard's future, trim it with a thin, flat barber's comb and barber's scissors. Run the comb through the part of the beard you want to trim and, holding it in place, snip off the hairs that protrude through the teeth of the comb.

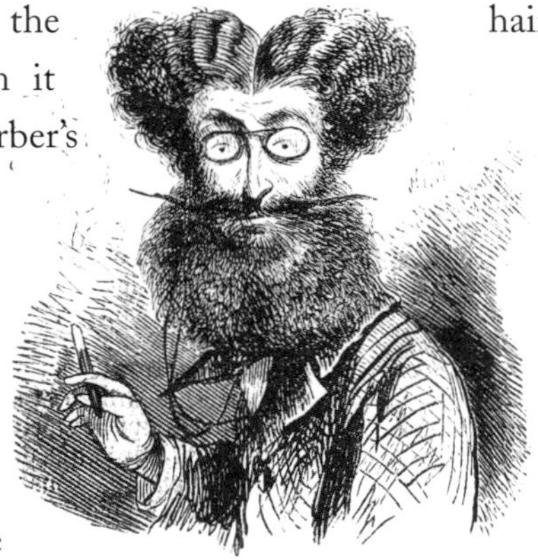

5. Unless your beard starts so far up your cheeks you look disquietingly apelike, leave that area alone. Don't shave it. Leave it natural. If there are some wild hairs up there, remove them individually with tweezers or nail scissors.

6. Wash your beard every time you wash your hair with a shampoo appropriate to your beard's hair type—which may be different from the hair on your head. After patting the beard dry, work a light moisturizer into your skin. Your beard may itch while it's growing in and it may even itch after it's done. Daily shampooing and time should remedy the situation.

Upon Shaving Off One's Beard
The scissors cut the
long-grown hair;
The razor scrapes the
remnant fuzz.
Small-jawed, weak-chinned,
big-eyed, I stare
At the forgotten boy I was.
John Updike

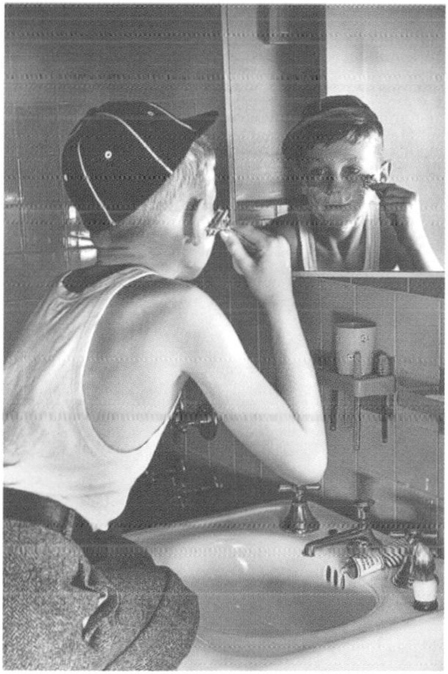

Four to six weeks into this experiment is long enough to know whether it's a success or a failure. If it's a failure—too patchy, too funky, too unpopular—lose it. Use clippers or scissor it off as close to the skin as you can. Then give your face a good soaking. If you have a heavy beard, use a preshave softener. Put a new blade in your razor, apply shaving cream—not foam, you need something you can work into the stubble—and if the first go-round doesn't do the job, rinse your face, put in a new blade, put on more shaving cream, and repeat the procedure.

One Size Does Not Fit All

After a month, you'll know where your beard comes in thick and where it comes in thin. You'll know if it's the same color as your hair. And you may want to give some thought to what style of beard goes with the shape of head you have. Since a beard covers the bottom of the face, it focuses attention on the top half, especially the eyes. If you have a long, thin face, a short, wide beard adds fullness. A rounded beard softens angularity and shortens a lantern jaw. If you have a chin even you can tell is weak, a squarish beard may help.

A beard will balance a receding hairline. Even a good mustache will provide a horizontal brake on all that forehead. But if you're totally bald or have a face shaped like a pie, a beard will call attention to both. Remember: Just because it looked good on that guy at the club doesn't mean it will look good on you. One size does not fit all.

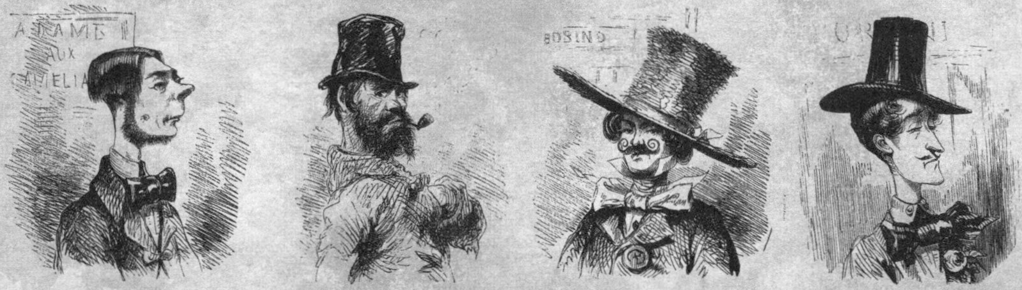

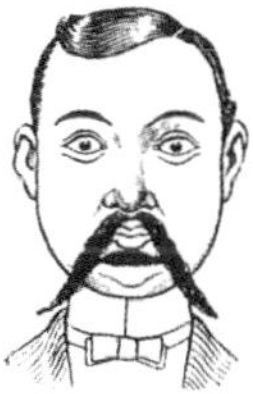

MR. ABELE

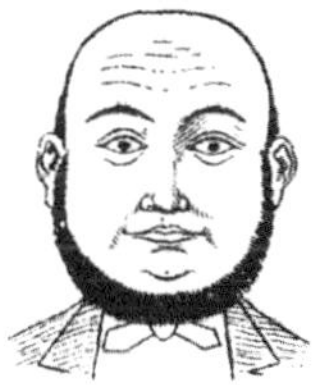

MR. COOK

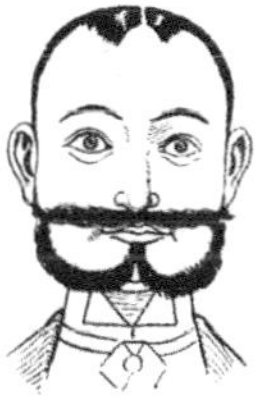

MR. BROWN

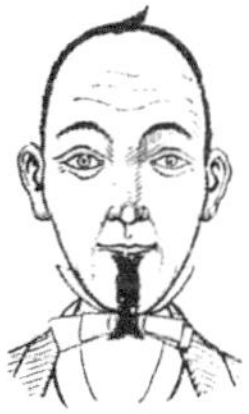

MR. IVINS

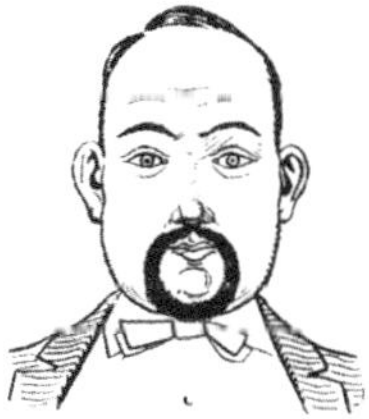

MR. OTTO

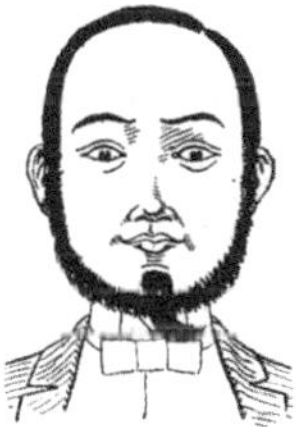

MR. QUILTER

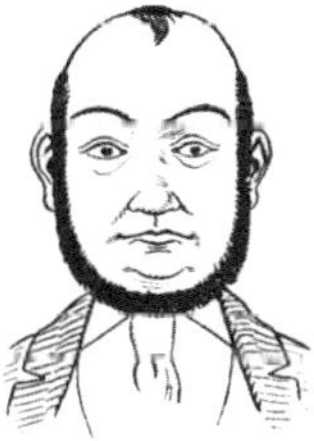

MR. UPWRIGHT

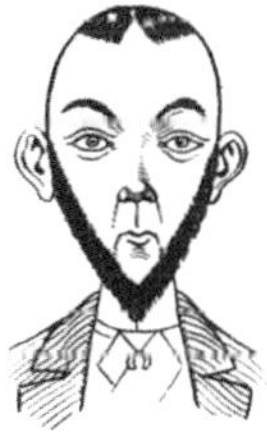

MR. VINCENT

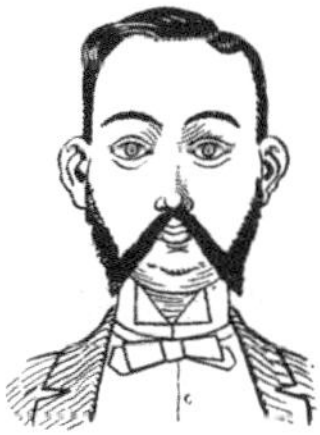

MR. WILCOX

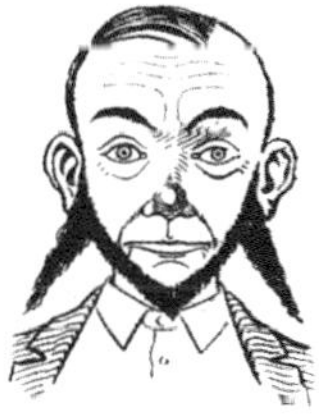

MR. MURPHY

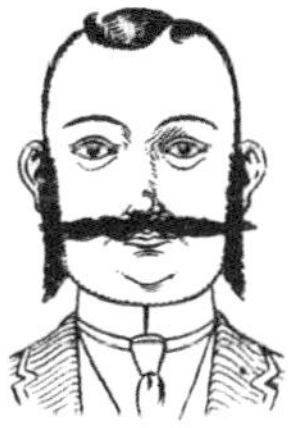

MR. HAPGOOD

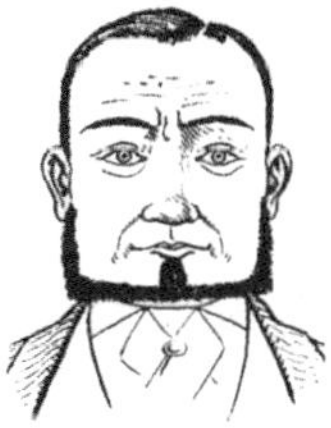

MR. ELVERSON

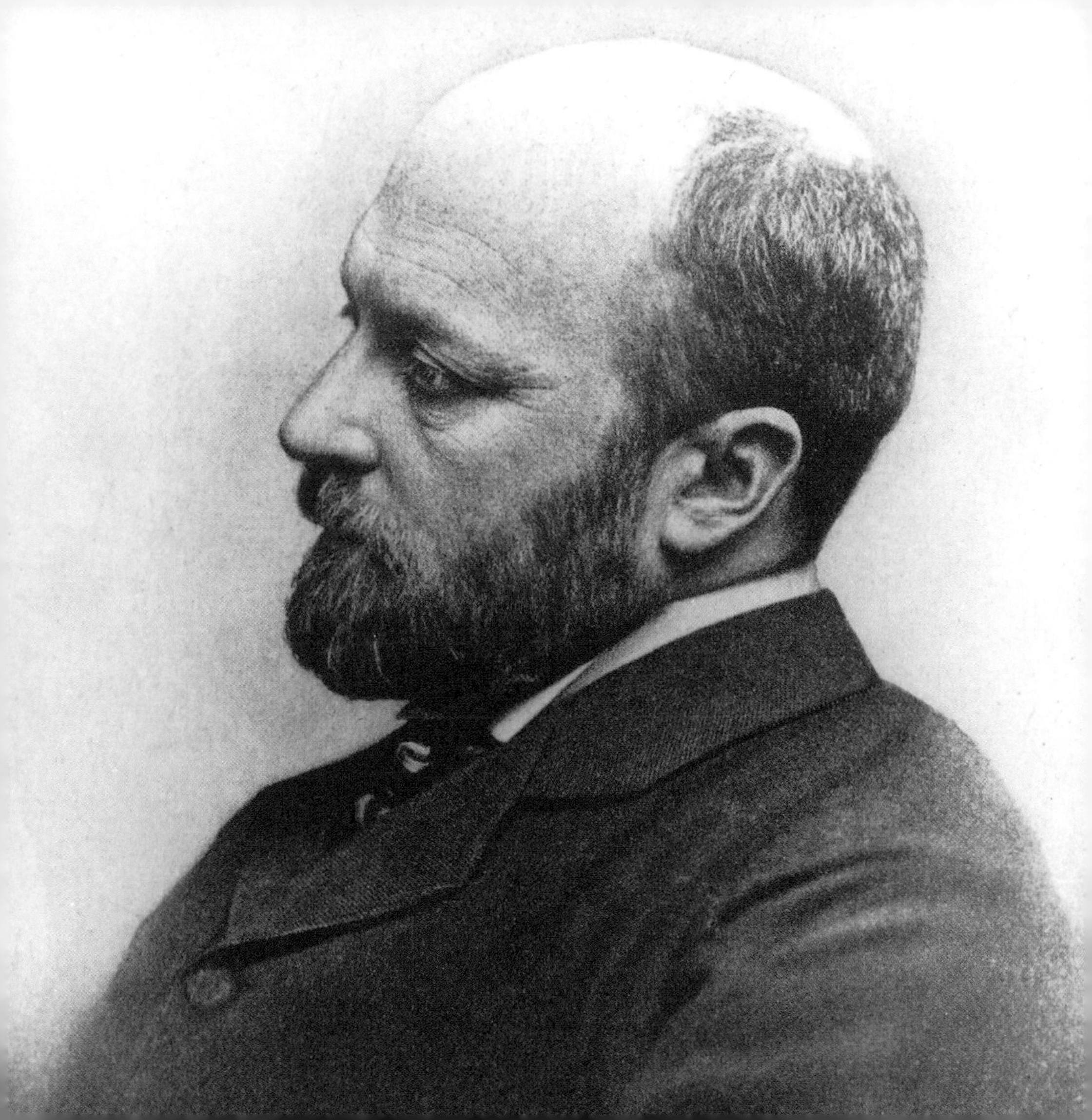

Changing Your Look

Growing a beard is one way a man can change his appearance. Shaving it off is another. The American novelist Henry James (1843–1916) had a beard from the time he was a young man until he was nearly sixty. He recorded his decision to get rid of it in a postcard to his brother:

Lamb House, Rye
May 12, 1900

Dearest William,

. . . No news with me save that I have totally shaved off my beard, unable to bear longer the increased hoariness of its growth: it had suddenly begun these three months since, to come out quite white and made me *feel* as well as look so old. Now, I feel *forty* and clean and light. . . .

Ever your,
Henry

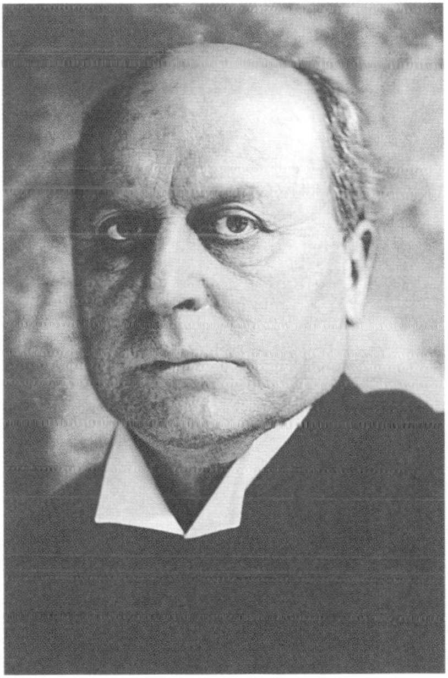

HOW TO SHAVE YOUR HEAD

Growing a beard requires patience and hope. Shaving your head requires nerve and existential optimism. If you don't like the way your beard has come in, you can undo in ten minutes the mistake that has taken a month to grow. If you don't like the way your newly bald head looks, reach for a hat and avoid mirrors.

A shaved head is a magnet for attention but it's practical too. You'll be spared falsely sympathetic references to the retreat of your hairline. No Indian waiter will ever have to ask if they got the saag paneer spicy enough. And without the side show of a head of hair, your individual features will be set off to better advantage: a prominent brow line, an off-center dimple, a goofy smile, sleepy eyes. So will the irregular lumps on the back of the skull, the Dumbo ears, and the tendency to pinheadedness.

There's something decisive and unfussy about a bare skull. Beard styles have names: spade, stiletto, goatee, soul patch, Horace Greeley, Vandyke. Hairstyles have names: pompadour, Caesar, horseshoe flattop, and the fade. Bald is . . . bald.

Right: Before he wore Darth Vader's helmet or became Bell Atlantic's voice, James Earl Jones was cool. Shaving his head was only part of it.

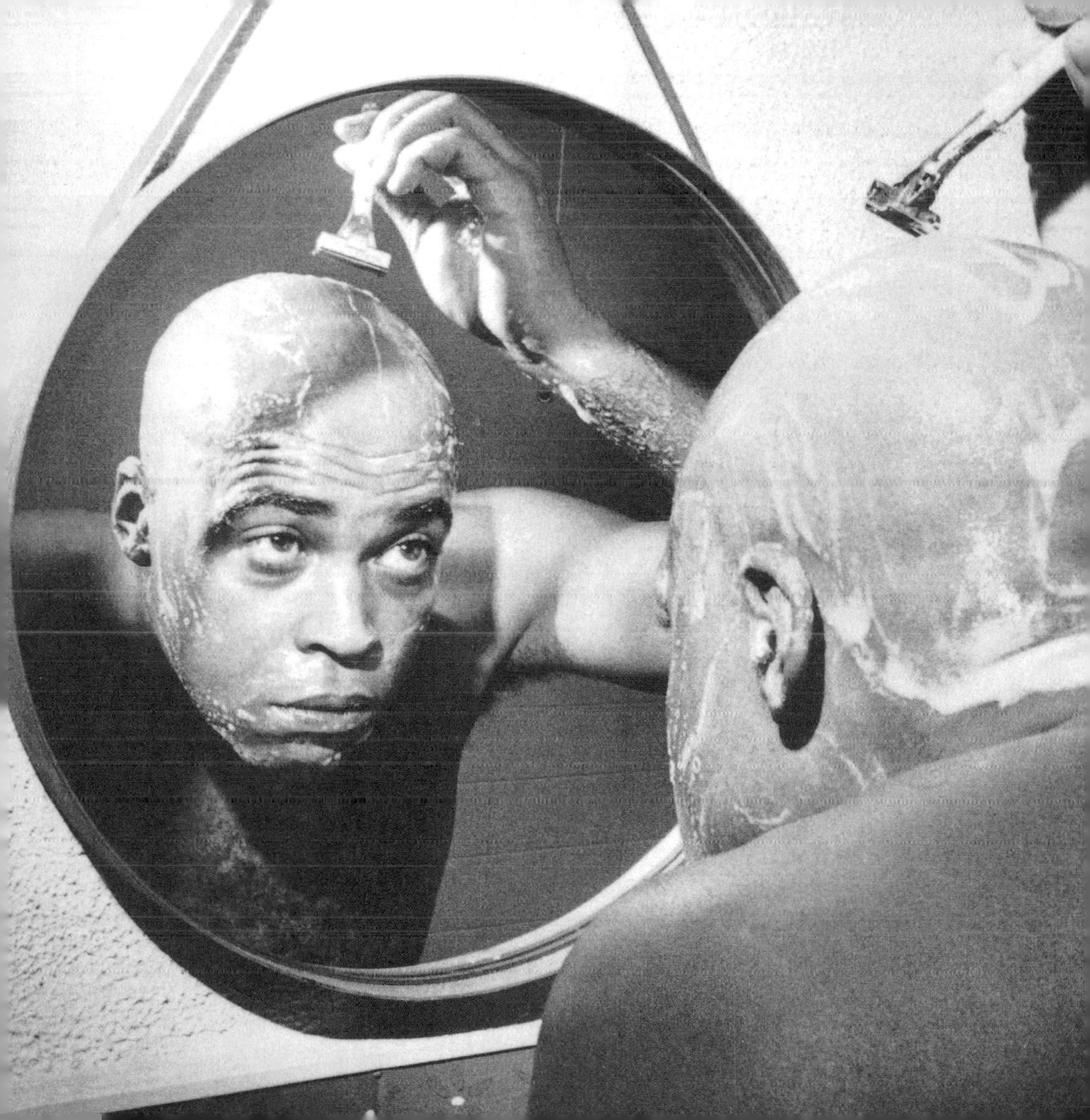

Discretionary Baldness

1. If you're starting with a good head of hair, the most efficient way to begin is with a buzz cut at the barbershop. Get your hair short enough so that you can remove what's left with a safety razor or an electric shaver. If you're a do-it-yourself kind of guy, do it yourself with electric clippers or shears. Clippers work better on dry hair than on wet hair; a damp scalp will create drag and may result in cuts and nicks.

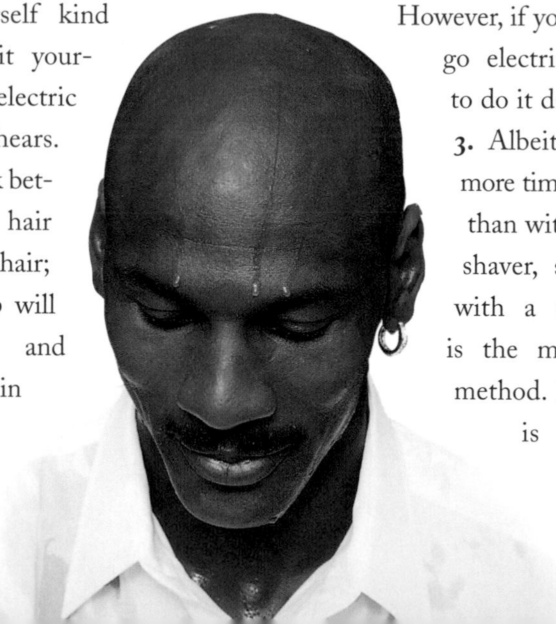

2. Once you've got all the hair off your skull, you have a couple of options for maintaining it that way. An electric shaver is fast, easy, and less likely than clippers to cause irritation with repeated use. Also, you get a closer cut. However, if you're going to go electric, you have to do it daily.

3. Albeit it is slightly more time-consuming than with an electric shaver, staying bald with a safety razor is the most popular method. If your goal is a pate as brilliant

as Daddy Warbucks', one that catches the light and throws it back, wet shaving is your only choice. Shower, apply shaving cream to your entire head, and commence shaving. Slowly and carefully, shave against the grain with a blade you've already used on your face a couple of times, using the shaving cream as an indicator of where you have to go next. Go over each spot once, rinsing the razor regularly so that it doesn't clog. Rinse your head and check for spots you've missed. It might not be a bad idea to finish off the process with an anti-residue shampoo, but a simple baby shampoo will do just as well. **4.** Pat your head dry, apply skin lotion to soothe your scalp and to maximize shine. Buffing it with a clean shoe cloth from time to time will maintain the shine as the day wears on.

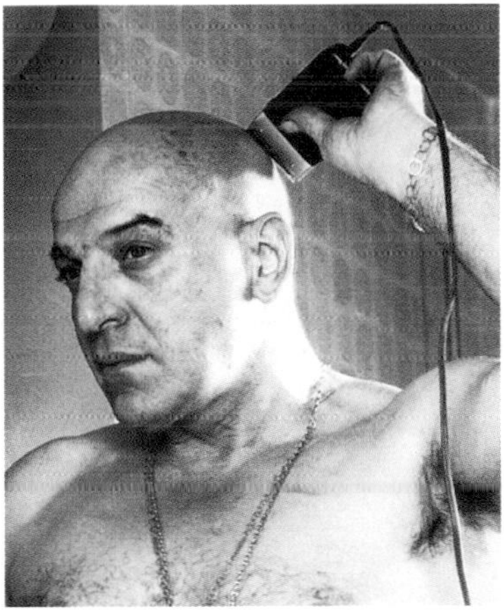

Above and left: In Kojak's day, only lovable eccentrics and Yul Brenner shaved their heads; the NBA and MTV made it mainstream.

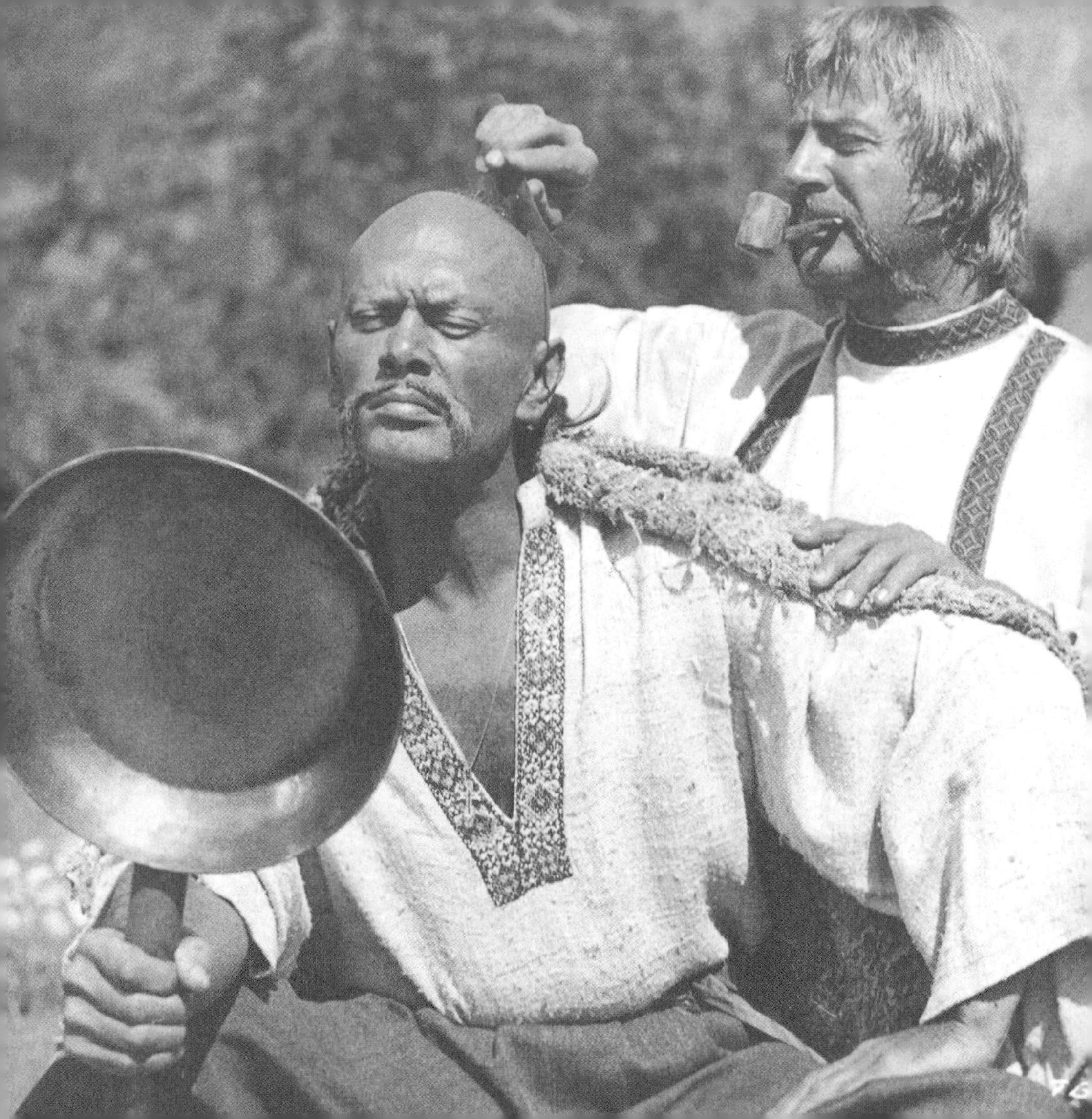

True, football players used to shave their shins and ankles so it wouldn't hurt when the tape they wrapped them with was removed. Cyclists shave their legs; some say it improves performance, some claim the nicks they get from flying gravel are less likely to get infected when there's no hair to trap the dirt, some do it because it looks cool.

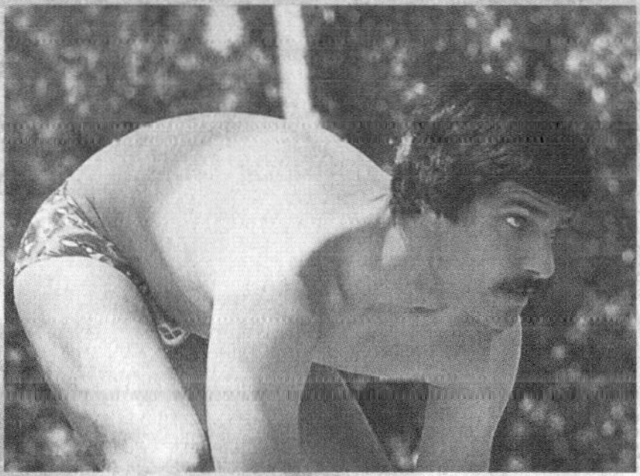

But just what kind of man shaves his entire body? A swimmer, supposedly to reduce drag in the fast lane but more practically to provide a psychological edge and, if the whole team shaves together before the big meet, a fraternal bond. A bodybuilder, because he wants to show off his definition, and body hair blurs the look. Transvestites going for verisimilitude shave; transvestites who think a hairy décolletage adds a certain je ne sais quoi do not.

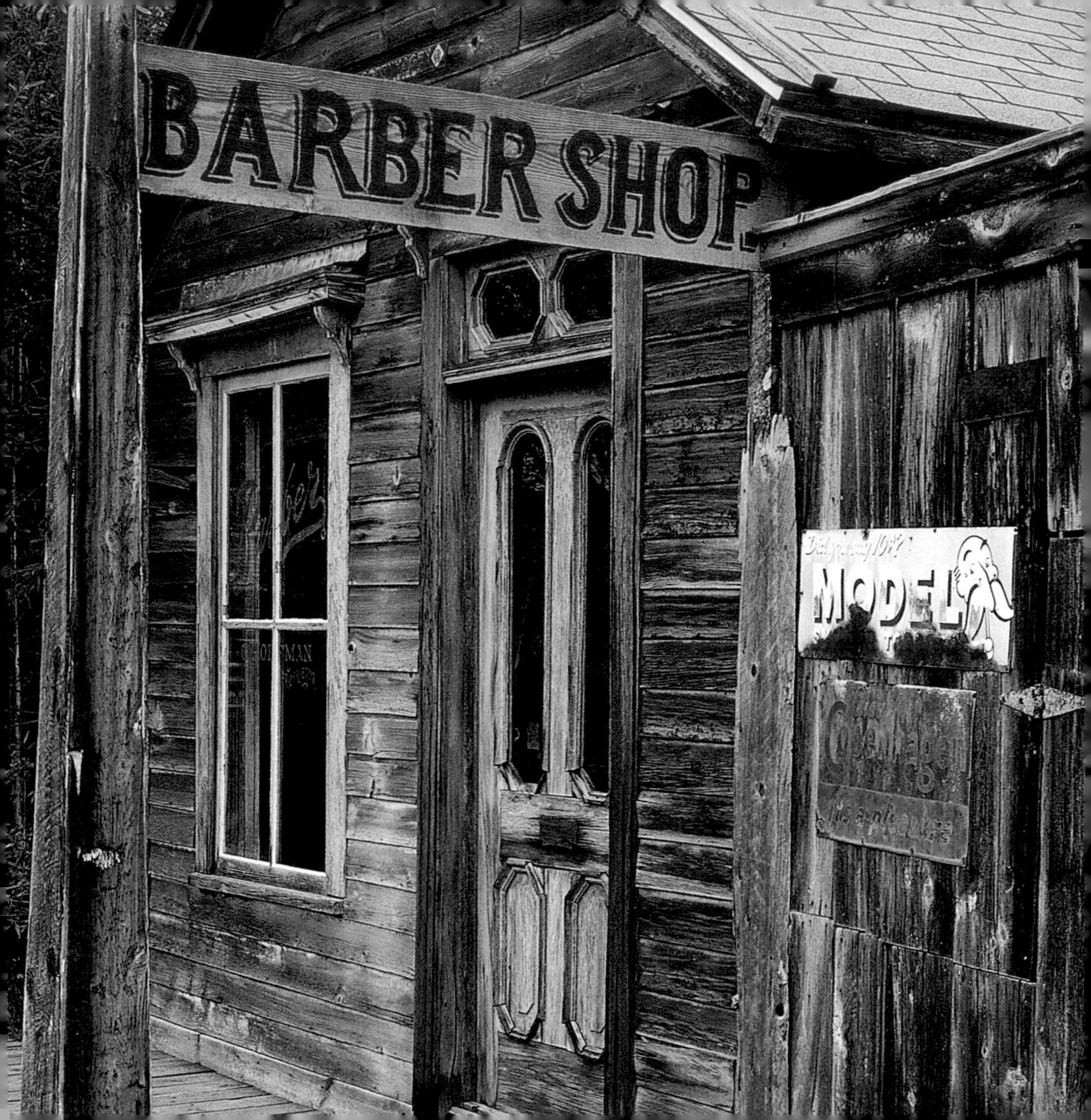
BARBER SHOP
MODEL

STRAIGHT RAZORS AND BARBERSHOP SHAVES

Talk in a barbershop is just as natural as silence in a mausoleum.
Charles De Zelmer

Hovering around the edges of the Zeitgeist is the memory that a straight or open (popularly known as a "cut-throat") razor produces a superior shave. In the hands of an experienced barber, it may. Unfortunately, the man in search of the ultimate shave will hunt long and hard before he finds a barber with the skill to administer it. Most men and women now cutting hair learn their trade in cosmetology schools where shaving is not taught. Fear of hepatitis and the HIV virus finished the revolution in masculine ritual that the advent of the safety razor began.

Formerly, neighborhood barbershops where a man could go for a regular shave were once as common as saloons. Now, it's a rare barber who even uses an open razor to square off a sideburn. Traditional barbershops—with their dog-eared copies of magazines like *Sports Afield* and *Police Gazette* splayed on chairs, a stuffed animal head mounted on the wall, and two or three men waiting their turns, chat-

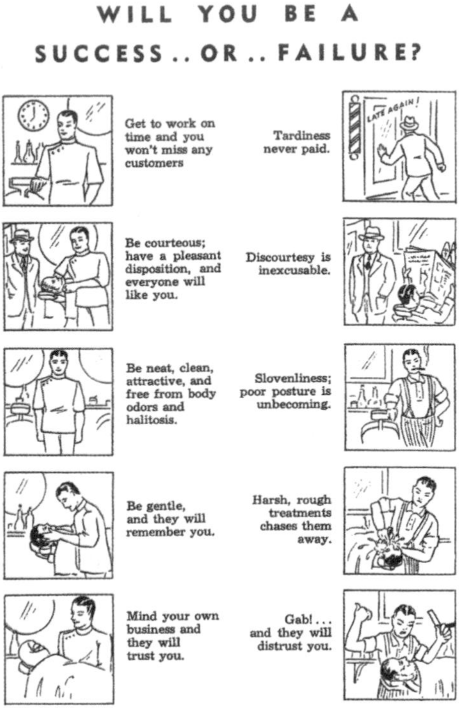
WILL YOU BE A
SUCCESS .. OR .. FAILURE?
Get to work on time and you won't miss any customers
LATE AGAIN!
Tardiness never paid.
Be courteous; have a pleasant disposition, and everyone will like you.
Discourtesy is inexcusable.
Be neat, clean, attractive, and free from body odors and halitosis.
Slovenliness; poor posture is unbecoming.
Be gentle, and they will remember you.
Harsh, rough treatments chases them away.
Mind your own business and they will trust you.
Gab! . . . and they will distrust you.

ting about high school football—still exist. But the ordinary pleasures of a scalp massage, steaming towel, and a finely honed razor skimming hot lather and whiskers off your chin, are gone for good.

Although the future is dim for traditional barbers, they can look back on a distinguished history. A few centuries ago, they did more than cut hair, trim beards, and give the occasional hot oil treatment. University-trained physicians compounded medicines, and barber-surgeons took care of the bloodier tasks healing was thought to require. In addition to giving shaves and haircuts they dressed wounds, lanced abscesses, and practiced the now abandoned arts of bloodletting, leeching, and cupping. Barbers in the American West pulled teeth throughout the 1800s and one St. Louis barber was still applying leeches as late as 1913.

To avoid romanticizing a vanishing institution, let's remember that barbers were necessary, but not necessarily well loved. "Barbers learn to shave by shaving fools" goes one proverb. But until the nineteenth century, a man had little choice. He could either risk his throat at the hands of a possibly inexperienced barber or trust himself to one he *knew* was inexperienced—himself.

Story of the Stripe

The red, white, and blue stripes on barber poles are a primer of barbering history. As a tradesman's symbol, the barber pole was used

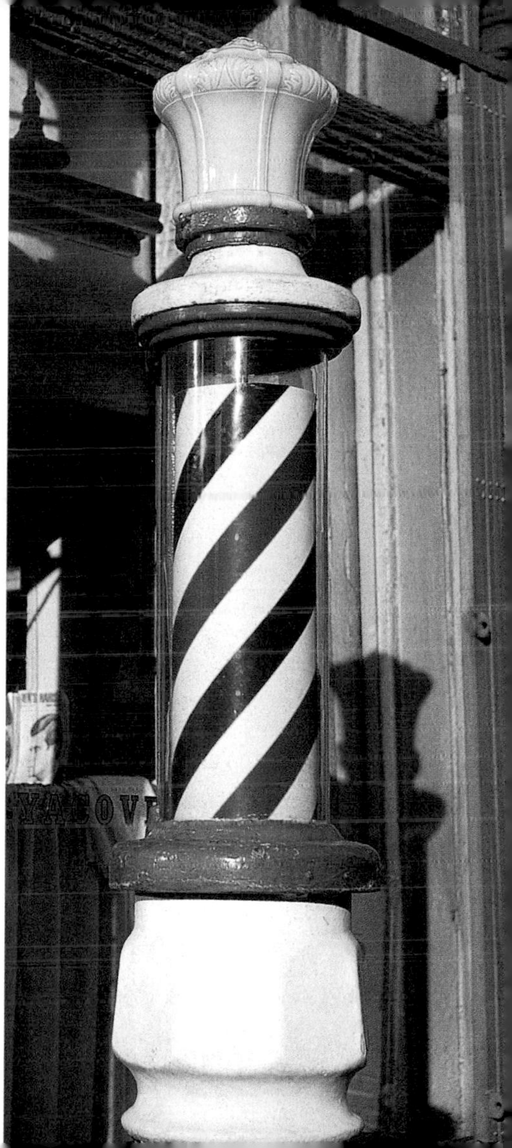

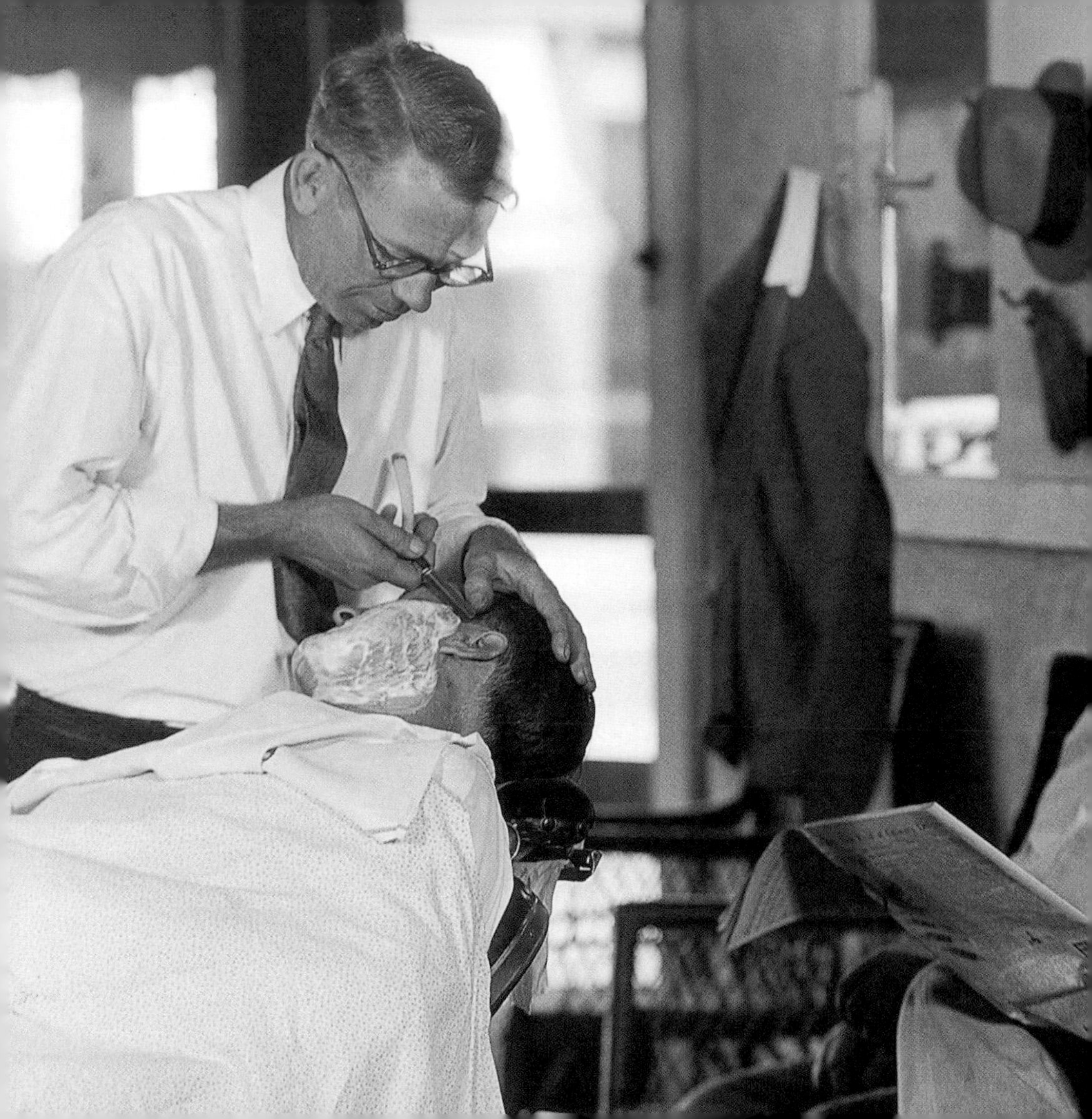

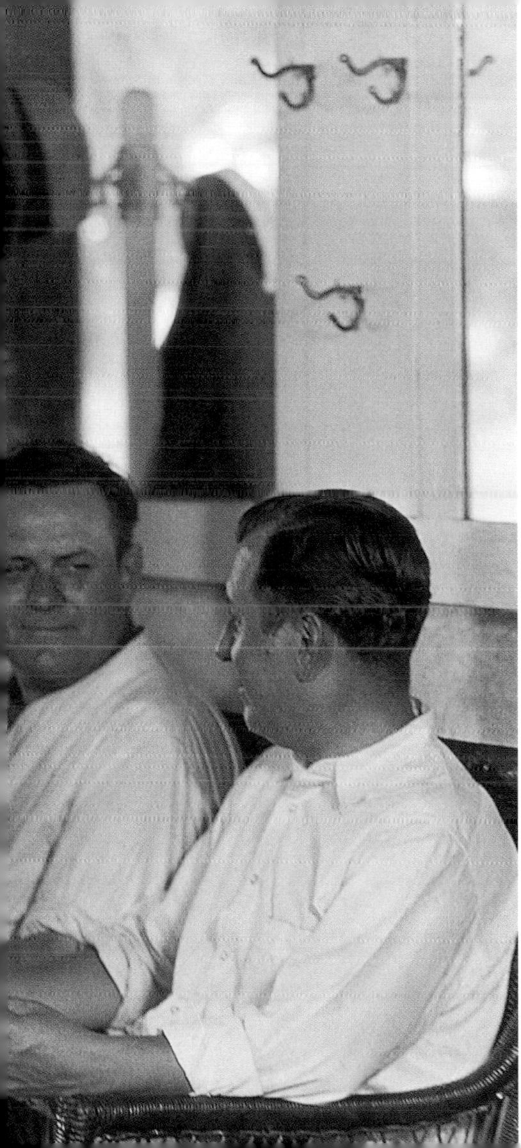

as early as the fourteenth century. A stout pole was set into the ground in front of a barber-surgeon's door; the patient sat in a chair in front of it, and while being lanced, cupped, or sewn up, he could grip the pole to better endure the pain. After the operation, the bloody bandages were hung from the pole to dry. Breezes would wrap them around the pole, whence the red spirals. Or so the story goes. This leaves us to wonder where the blue spirals come from.

The professions of barber and surgeon have separated and merged several times over the course of time. One folk explanation for the barber pole's stripes has it that surgeons appropriated the bloodier, red-striped pole as their professional symbol while the barbers invented a blue-striped one for theirs. When the professions came back together, so did the two separate poles—and voilà, red, white, and blue. Still another explanation is that the red represents arterial blood, the blue venous blood, and the white the shop's high standards of hygiene or the bandage itself.

Given the fact that barber-surgeons flourished centuries before the invention of anesthesia and bore more of a resemblance to butchers than to their present-day descendants, the survival of the barber pole as a tradesman's symbol is remarkable. Equally remarkable is the demand for either new or refurbished barber poles. And at auctions of American folk art, an older specimen can fetch a price equal to half a modern barber's annual salary.

Writers on Barbershops

Shaves Around the World

. . . I thought of all the barbers of my career. . . . New York barbers, who, rendered callous by the harsh and complex splendor of their catacombs, take hold of your head as if it was your foot, or perhaps a detachable wooden sphere. I like Denmark because there some of the barbers' shops have a thin ascending jet of water whose summit just caresses the bent chin, which after shaving is thus laved without either the repugnant British sponge or the clumsy splashing necessary in France and Italy.

French barbers are far better than the English. They greet you kindly when you enter their establishments, and invariably create in

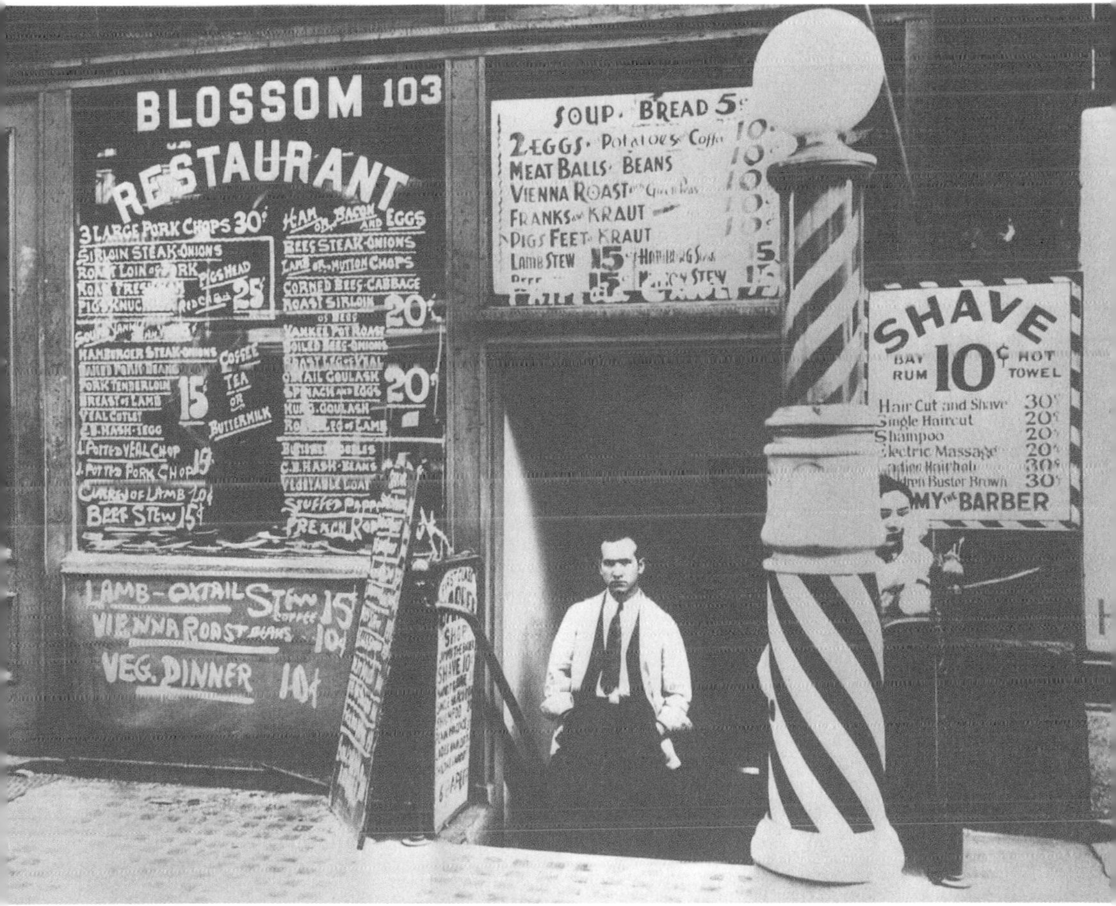
BLOSSOM 103
RESTAURANT
3 LARGE PORK CHOPS 30¢
SIRLOIN STEAK-ONIONS
PIGS HEAD
25¢
HAM OR BACON AND EGGS
BEEF STEAK-ONIONS
LAMB OR MUTTON CHOPS
CORNED BEEF-CABBAGE
ROAST SIRLOIN OF BEEF
20¢
YANKEE POT ROAST
BOILED BEEF-ONIONS
20¢
HAMBURGER STEAK-ONIONS
PORK TENDERLOIN
BREAST OF LAMB
VEAL CUTLET
15¢
COFFEE TEA OR BUTTERMILK
BEEF STEW 15¢
LAMB-OXTAIL STEW 15
VIENNA ROAST BEANS 10¢
VEG. DINNER 10¢
SOUP. BREAD 5¢
2 EGGS. POTATOES COFFEE 10¢
MEAT BALLS. BEANS
VIENNA ROAST
FRANKS AND KRAUT
PIGS FEET AND KRAUT
LAMB STEW 15¢
SHAVE
BAY RUM 10¢ HOT TOWEL
Hair Cut and Shave 30¢
Single Haircut 20¢
Shampoo 20¢
Electric Massage 20¢
Children Buster Brown 30¢
BARBER

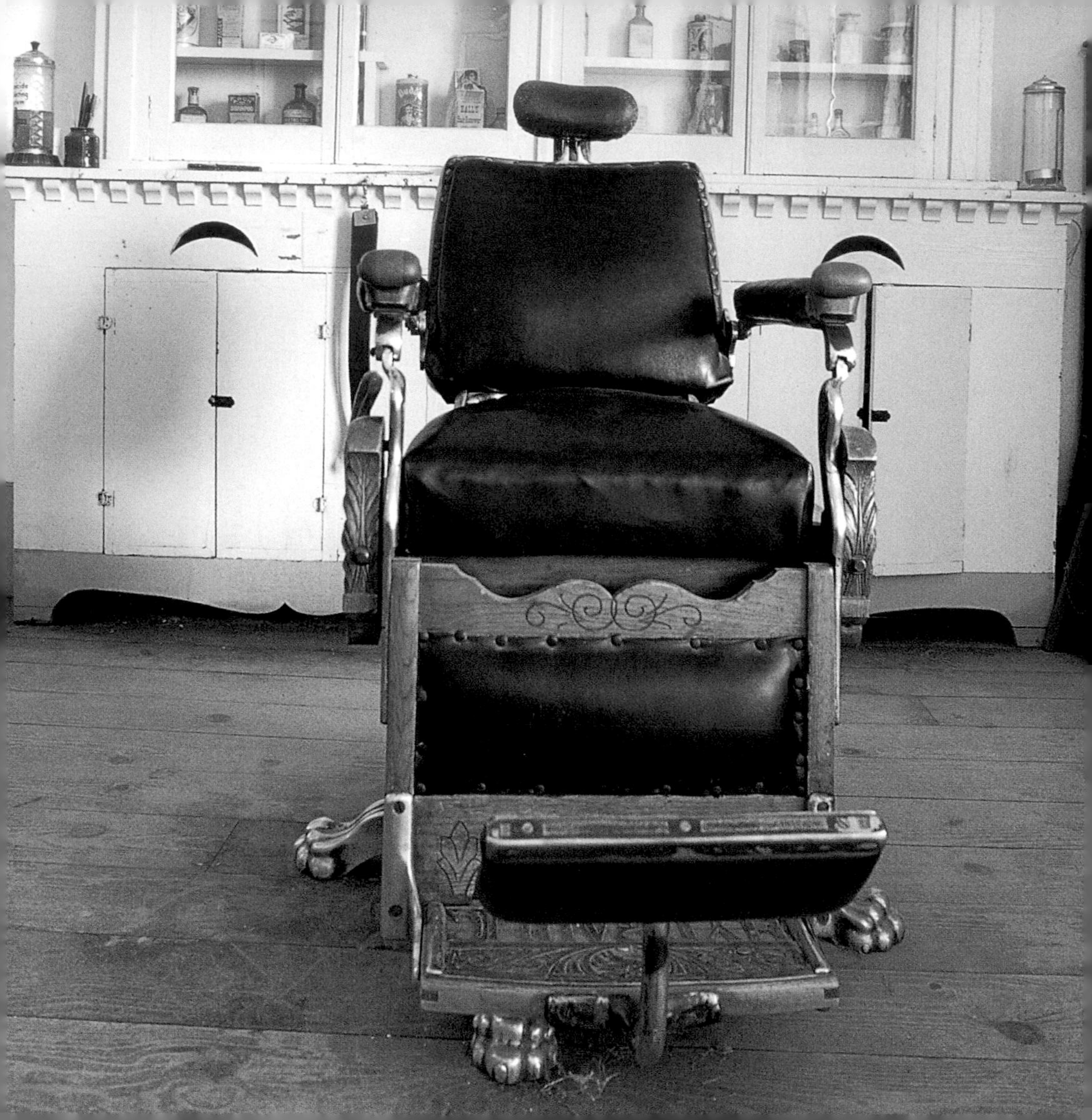

you the illusion that you will not have to wait. For years I knew very well indeed the sole barber of a very small French village. The man was in his excellent shop fourteen hours a day seven days a week. He had one day's holiday every year Easter Monday, when he went to Paris for the day.

Arnold Bennett

My Father's Mug

Clarkie's shop was in [the] Lyceum Hall block, one flight up—a huge room, with a single green upholstered barber's chair between the windows, where you could sit and watch the town go by below you. The room smelled pungently of bay rum. Barber shops don't smell of bay rum anymore. Around two sides were ranged many chairs and an old leather couch. The chair-arms were smooth and black with the rubbing of innumerable hands and elbows, and behind them, making a dark line along the wall, were the marks where the heads of the sitters rubbed as they tilted back. Nor can I forget the spittoons—large, shallow boxes, two feet square—four of them, full of sand. On a third side of the room stood the basin and water-taps, and beside them a large black-walnut cabinet, full of shelves. The shelves were full of mugs, and on every mug was a name, in gilt letters, generally Old English. Those mugs were a town directory of our leading citizens. My father's mug

Left: A barber's chair in Columbia, California

was on the next to the top shelf, third from the end on the right. The sight of it used to thrill me, and at twelve I began surreptitiously to feel my chin, to see if there were any hope of my achieving a mug in the not too distant future.

Above the chairs, the basin, the cabinet, hung pictures. I know not what has become now of Clarkie or his shop. Doubtless they have gone the way of so many pleasantly flavored things of our vanished New England.

Oliver Wendell Holmes

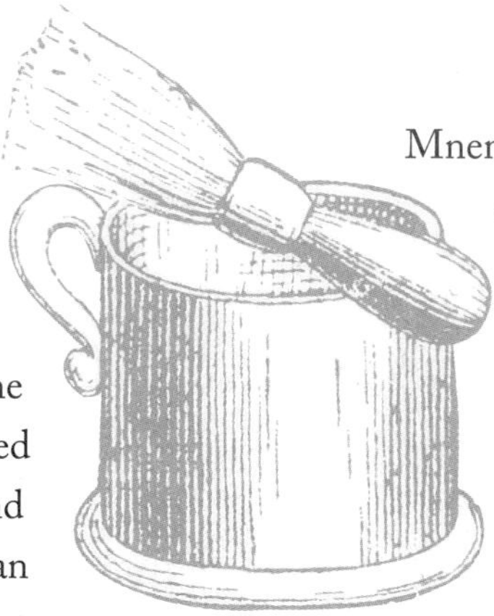

Alexandria Seer

Mnemjian's Babylonian barber's shop was on the corner of Fuad I and Nebi Daniel and here every morning Pombal lay down beside me in the mirrors. We were lifted simultaneously and swung smoothly down in to the ground wrapped like dead Pharaohs, only to reappear at the same instant on the ceiling spread out like specimens. White cloths had been spread over us by a small black boy while in a great Victorian mustache cup the barber thwacked up his dense and sweet-smelling lather before applying it in direct considered brush-strokes to our cheeks. The first covering complete, he surrendered his task to an assistant while he went to the great strop hanging among the flypapers on the end wall of the shop and began to sweeten the edge of an English razor.

Little Mnemjian is a dwarf with a violet eye that has never lost its childhood. He is the Memory man, the archives of the city. If you should wish to know the ancestry or income of the most casual passer-by you have only to ask him; he will recite the details in a sing-song voice as he strops his razor and tries it upon the coarse black hair of his forearm. What he does not know he can find out in a matter of moments. Moreover he is as well briefed in the living as in the dead; I mean this in the literal sense, for the Greek Hospital employs him to shave and lay out its victims before they are committed to the undertakers—a task which he performs with relish tinged by racial unction. His ancient trade embraces the two worlds, and some

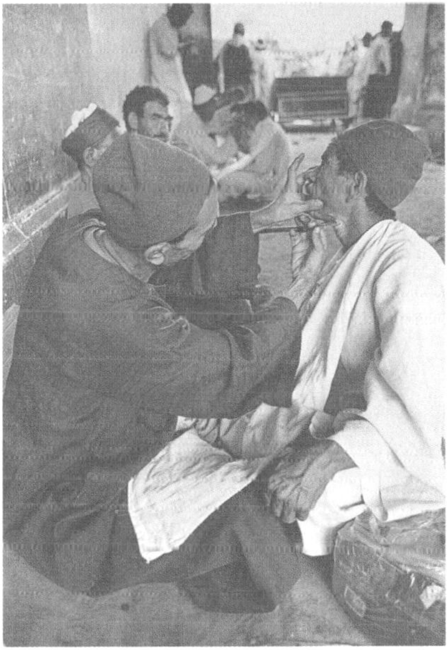

Above: A man can get as good a shave out of doors as in the poshest tonsorial parlor. Here, a street barber plies his trade (Cairo, *circa* 1988).

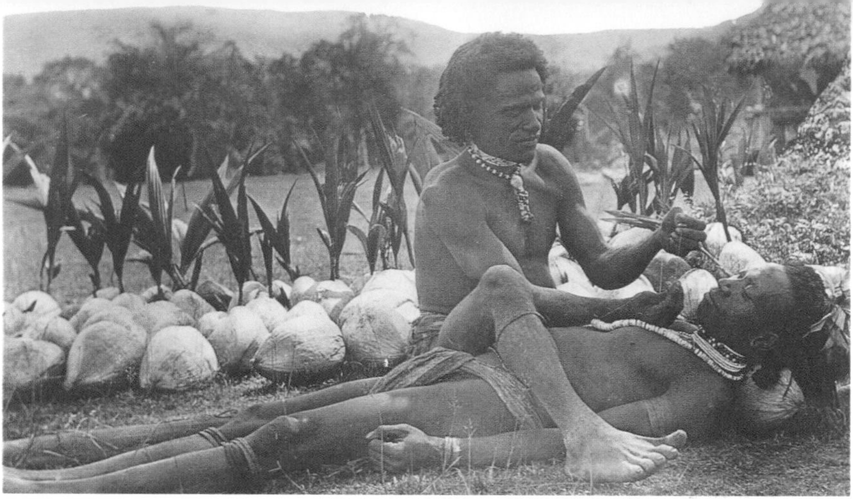

Above: Pulling out each hair with a loop of twisted fiber assured a high pain-efficiency ratio on the New Guinea Coast in this early twentieth century photo.

of his best observations begin with the phrase: "As so-and-so said to me with *his last breath*. . . ."

While he works with a razor his eyes dim out and his features become as expressionless as a bottle. His fingers travel as coolly upon our live faces as they do upon those of the fastidious and (yes, lucky) dead."

Lawrence Durrell, *Justine*

Shaved with a String in Egypt

The barber was about eighty years old and he had only one good eye. He clenched a spool of string in his teeth, wrapped the thread around two outstretched fingers on one hand and made it taut by pulling it with the other. Then he leaned down close enough to kiss me and waved his hands over my face. The one-eyed barber and his thread ripped my hairs, one by one, out by the root.

It was more painful than having wisdom teeth yanked, but I could not leave the chair. It was, after all, an act of hospitality. And suddenly the shop was filled with men, craning to watch.

There are 30,000 whiskers on a man's face. The barber wanted to remove every one of mine.

"Kif halek?" one of the men called out. "How are you?"

"El hamdehrella," I cried. "I'm well, thank God."

There was deep laughter, a communion among men. Somebody brought me a falafel. The barber stopped. I ate slowly, thankful for the reprieve. An hour later, when the barber finished, my skin felt like a satin slip. . . ."

Cal Fussman

Getting Shaved in Turkey

I got my first shave in a barber's chair some years ago in the Turkish seaside town of Marmaris from a ten-year-old who was minding the shop for the owner. . . .

My artery emerged unsevered, but it was one of the most painful twenty minutes I ever spent. It felt as if the boy had peeled off the top layer of my skin, and then gone back to remove the next one down. In his favor, it was the best shave I have ever had—for 48 hours my face was as smooth as a cue ball—and the process left no actual blood.

When I returned to Turkey for a visit last year, I decided once again to put myself in the hands of a professional. This time I went in the company of a Turkish friend . . . to a hole in the wall barbershop with two chairs, decorated by a calendar with a girl in a substantial bikini, and the inevitable portrait of Kemal Ataturk.

The first thing I learned, thanks to my friend's translating, was that the ideal shave in Turkey is called *sinek aydi*—so smooth that a fly would slide off—and that there are two kinds. If the barber goes against the grain of your beard, you get the closest shave, but it hurts like hell. This is what the ten-year-old had been selling. If he goes with the grain, it won't hurt, though you will show a five o'clock shadow—five o'clock of the day after.

The barber, who looked like a kindly Hafez Assad, began by notching a razor blade and fitting it into a tortoiseshell handle. Then he lathered me up. After each sweep of the blade, he wiped the foam onto the base of the thumb of his opposite hand; every three or four strokes, he shook the buildup into the sink. He worked quickly and carefully, and when he was finished, he did it all over again, lest a fly find a foothold. When he was done, lotion, cream and powder went on my face in successive applications, like coats of paint on a car. For the climax, he took a long Q-tip, dipped it in flaming Sterno and flicked it deftly in each ear, like a conductor tapping a baton, to singe the little hairs. It cost about the equivalent of two bits.

Richard Brookhiser

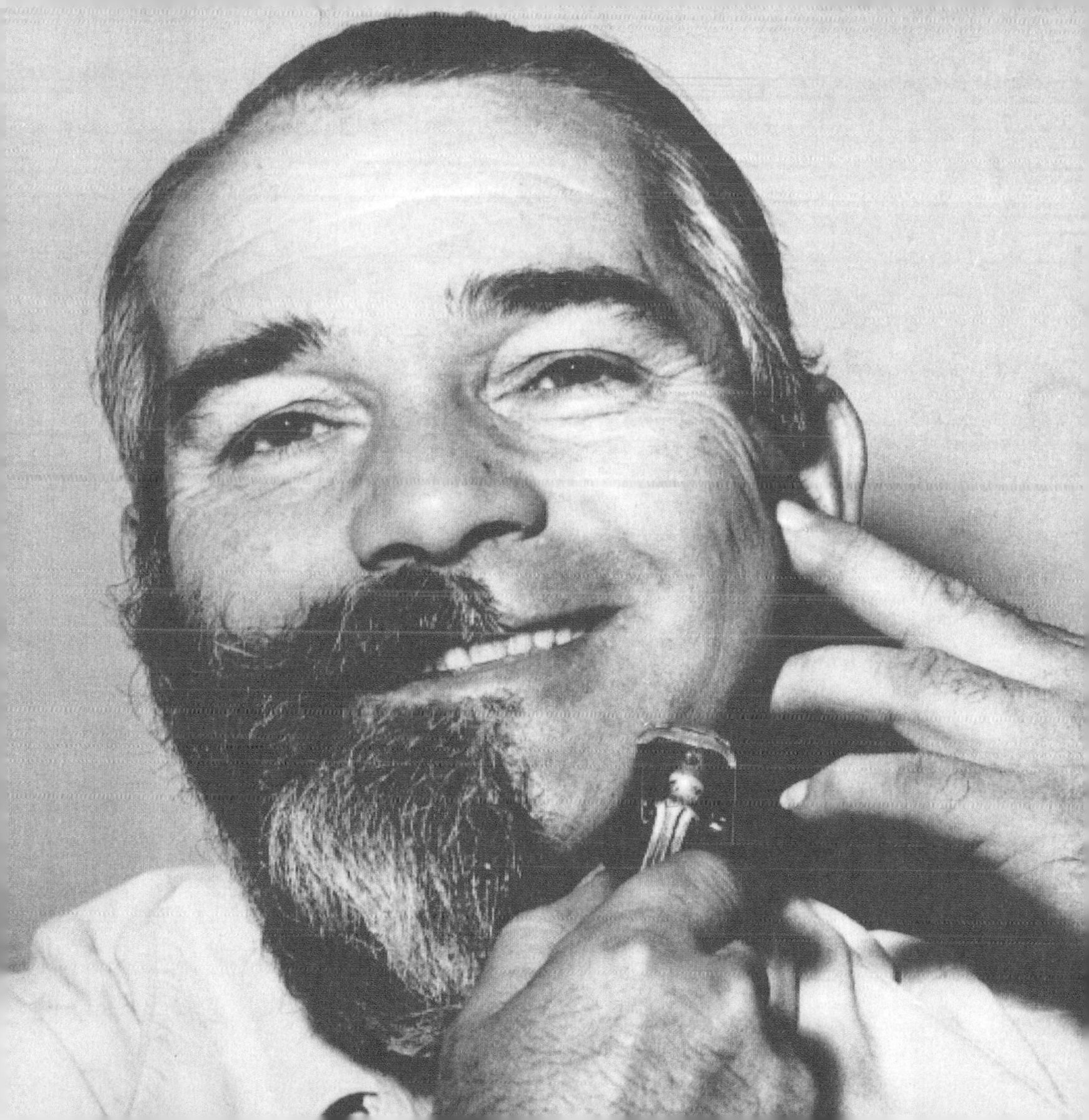

THE MARCH OF PROGRESS

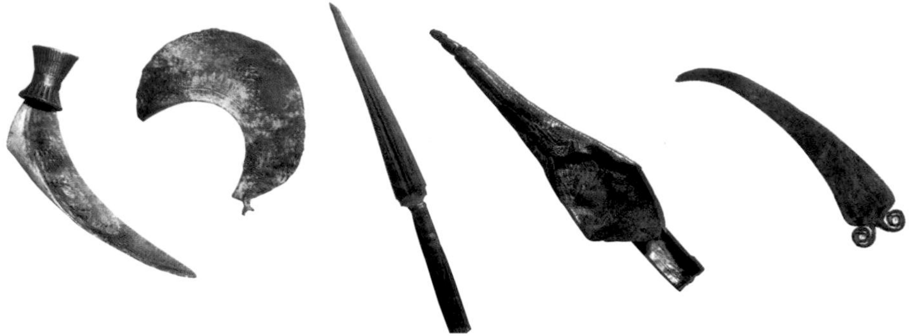

10000 B.C. Cave drawings depict men with short beards and beardless men. Sharpened flints and crude tweezers are the likely tools for shaving and trimming.

4000 B.C. Razorlike implements made of copper alloy appear in Egypt.

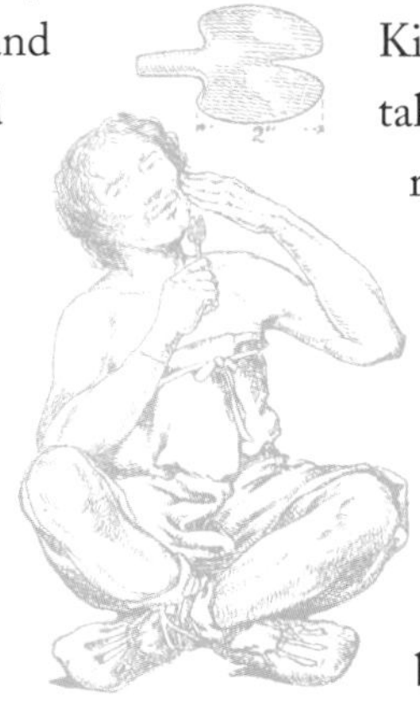

1567–1320 B.C. New Kingdom bronze razors take a better edge and replace copper razors.

1000 B.C. Iron replaces bronze for tools and weapons.

Human sacrifices preserved in Danish bogs are clean-shaven.

323 B.C. Alexander the Great orders his troops to shave.

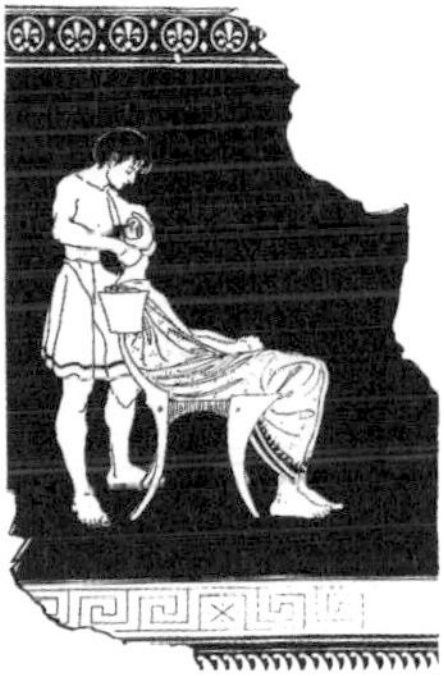

296 B.C. Greek barbers are brought from Sicily to Rome. Until now, the Romans considered shaving an effeminate Greek affectation.

200 B.C. The Roman legions use pumice stones to sand off their beards; civilians offer themselves up to the barber's blade only once a month.

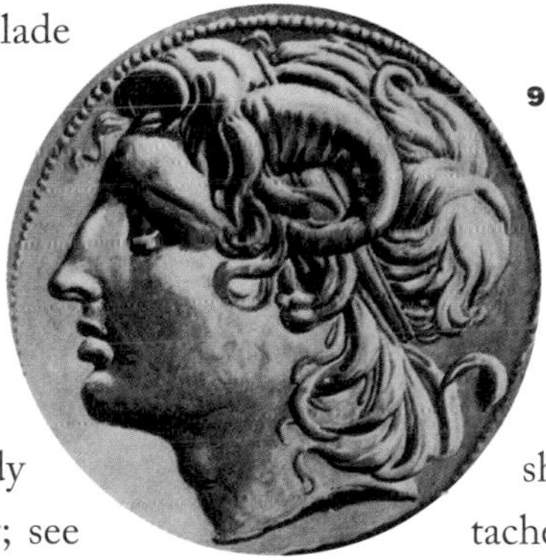

A.D. 10 In his *Ars Amatoria*, Ovid gives the following advice to young men: "Let exercise your body brown:/ Don't slobber; see your teeth are clean/ Your hair well cut and brushed quite down:/ Your cheeks close shaved with razor keen."

330-63 After generations of government by clean-shaven Christian generals, the Roman emperor Julian grows his beard to let people know that a pagan philosopher is now on the throne.

980 Full beards come back into fashion after centuries in which most rulers were clean-shaven or had, at most, a short beard or a mustache. After Otto III, the

Holy Roman emperors are depicted with beards.

1031 Canon 7 of the Council of Bourges states that all clerics "who minister within the holy church should have an ecclesiastical tonsure, that is, a shaven beard and

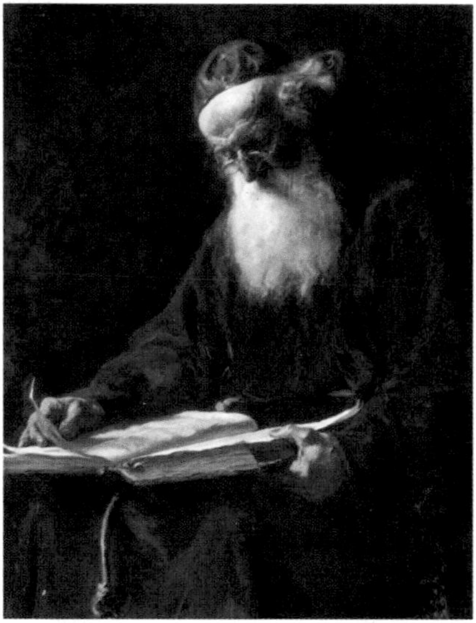

a circle on the head." Tonsure is to the Middle Ages what the clerical collar would become in modern times.

1066 In the Battle of Hastings, Anglo-saxon king Harold seriously underestimates Norman forces because of a simple misunderstanding on the part of his spies in France, who assumed any man with neither beard nor mustache was a priest.

1163 A papal decree forbids the clergy to commit the sacrilege of shedding blood. Monks who are required to do regular bloodletting turn these duties over to the barbers.

1361 French barbers and surgeons form a guild.

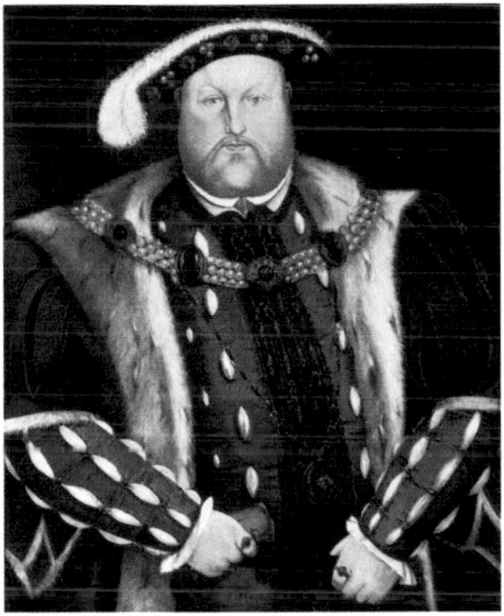

Above: Henry VIII

1462 Edward IV grants English barbers a charter as a trade guild. Henry VIII amalgamates them with the university-trained surgeons in 1541, but with a charter stipulating that the only surgery they can perform is bloodletting and pulling teeth. The surgeons are forbidden to practice shaving.

1610–43 Louis XIII occupies the French throne. As he loses his hair, the powdered wig becomes popular; for the next two hundred years, facial hair is out of favor.

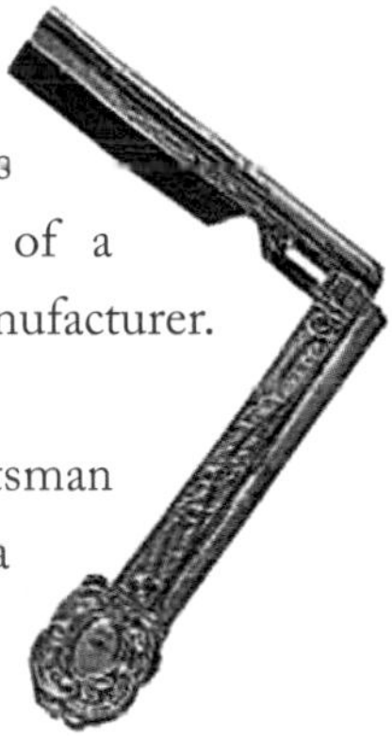

1680 First appearance of the narrow-bladed folding straight razor is made in the records of a Sheffield (England) manufacturer.

1740 Benjamin Huntsman invents cast steel—a harder, finer-grained steel better able to take and hold an edge.

1769 Jean-Jacques Perret, a cutler, publishes *La Pogonotomie*, which proposes the relatively new idea that men should learn to shave them-

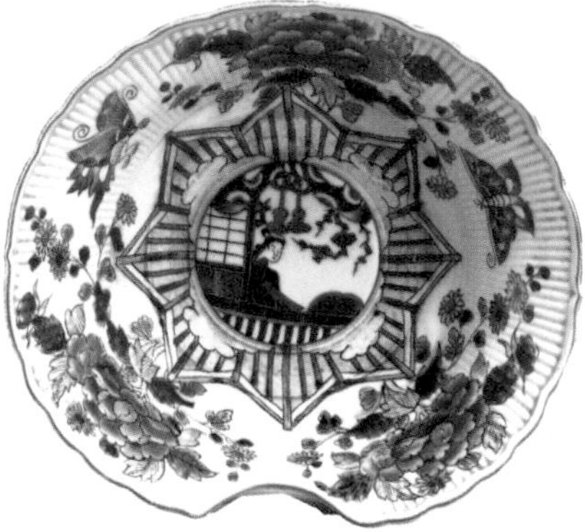

Above: Imari barber's bowl, eighteenth century

selves—not a simple task because of razor design. Since it is wide at one end and tapering into a handle, with no shoulder separating the blade from the tang, it is easy for the finger to slip onto the cutting edge.

1776 The signers of the Declaration of Independence are all clean-shaven, unless we count Edward Rutledge of South Carolina. (Mr. Rutledge combs his rather long hair over his forehead and cheeks so it can be seen in front of his ears, but he is technically as clean-shaven as his co-signatories.)

1800s Barber's Itch, an age-old infection transmitted by dirty brushes and tools, continues to be the bane of barbershops throughout the century.

1820 Michael Faraday adds a tiny quantity of silver to the cast steel

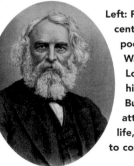

Left: Popular nineteenth-century American poet Henry Wadsworth Longfellow lost his wife in a fire. Burned in his attempt to save her life, he grew a beard to cover the scars.

blade; progress in metallurgy enables razor design to evolve, allowing for better control of the instrument.

1847 Londoner William Henson has the ingenious idea of placing a razor's handle perpendicular to its blade, thus creating the first "hoe-type" razor.

1850s English soldiers return from the Crimean War sporting beards; soon every self-respecting middle-class man sprouts one.

1861 Civil War hero General Ambrose E. Burnside affects whiskers in front of the ears and along the cheeks; they are known as "burnsides" until folk etymology decides that since they are worn on the sides, they should be called "sideburns."

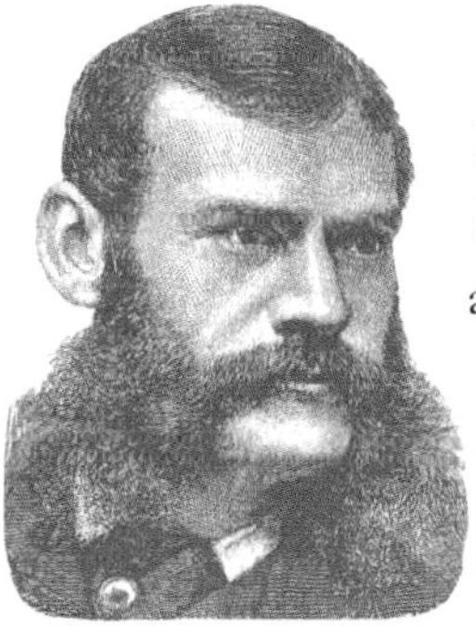

Above: In the 1890's, what we call sideburns were still known as burnsides.

Below: Gustave Flaubert earns the nickname Abu Chanab (Father of the Mustache) during his travels through Egypt.

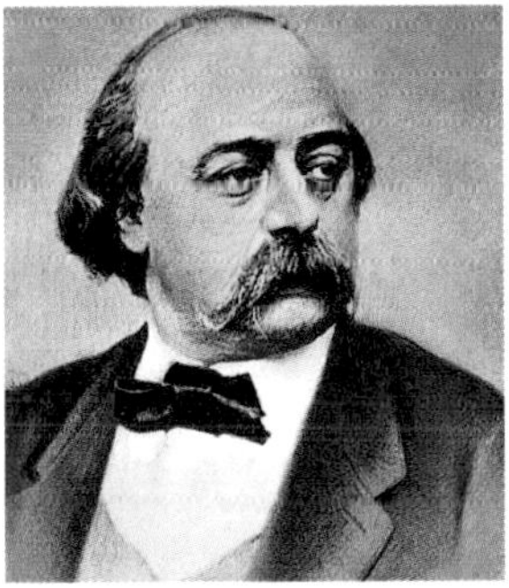

1862 The extravagant sideburns known in England as muttonchops are called dundrearys in the United States, in honor of a character, Lord Dundreary, in the play President Lincoln was watching the night he was shot.

Below: Men who patronize barbers, on Fleet Street or Main Street, are more likely to be talked to death than decapitated.

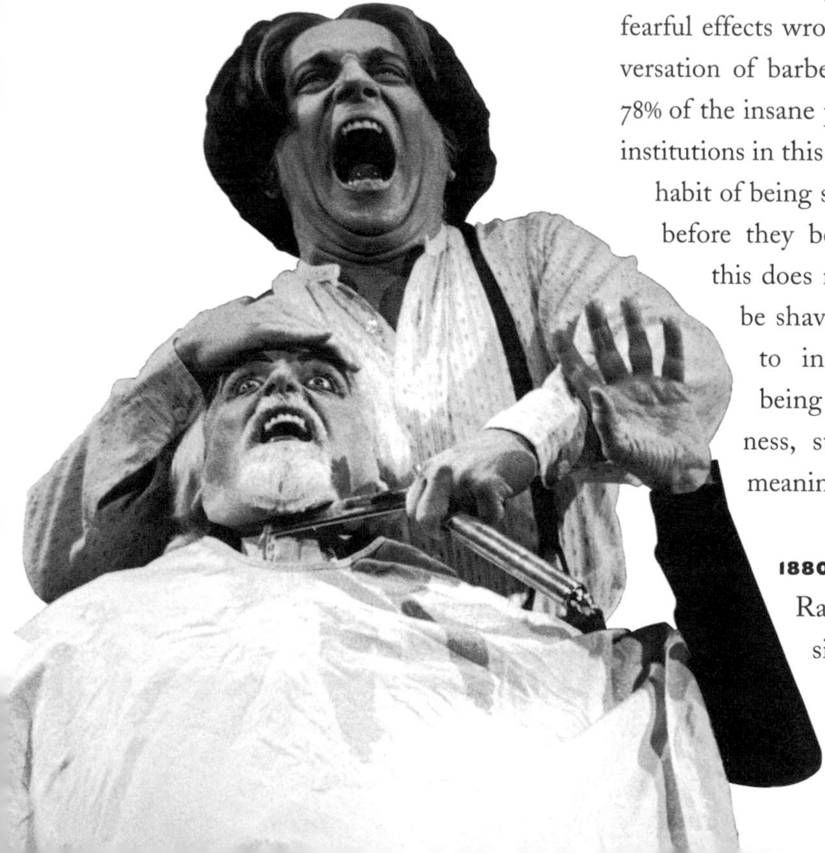

1879 *The New York Times* carries the article headlined BARBERS TERRORIZE PUBLIC: "The records of our insane asylums show the fearful effects wrought by the conversation of barbers. No less than 78% of the insane patients in public institutions in this State were in the habit of being shaved by barbers before they became insane. If this does not mean that to be shaved by a barber is to incur the risk of being talked into madness, statistics have no meaning."

1880 Star Safety Razor, featuring a single-edge blade in a holder that is attached to a

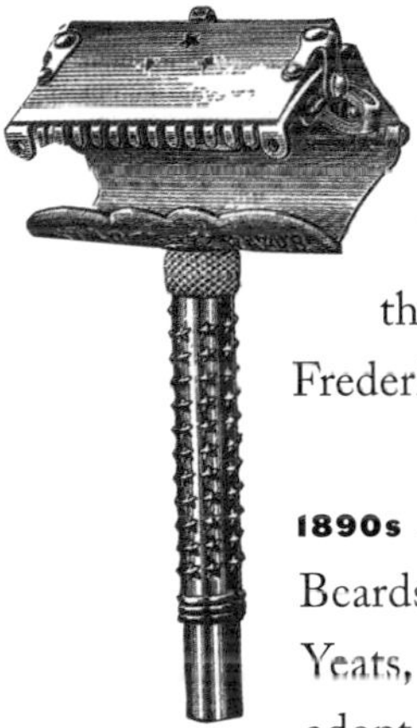

hoe-type handle, is patented in the United States by the brothers Otto and Frederick Kampfe.

1890s Artists like Aubrey Beardsley, William Butler Yeats, and Oscar Wilde adopt a clean-shaven look as a specific mark of protest against the bearded Philistine middle-class.

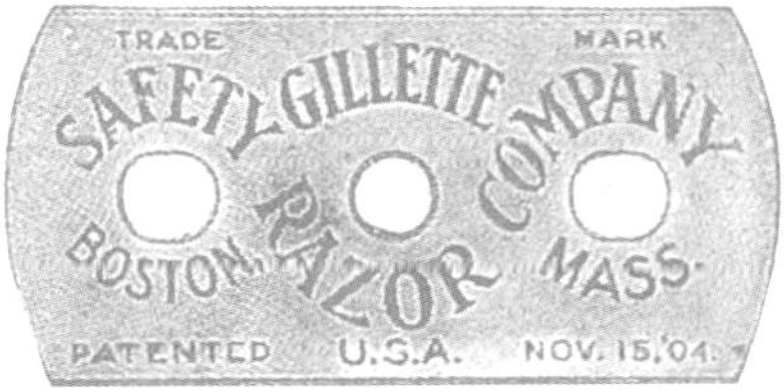

1895 Visionary entrepreneur King Camp Gillette comes up with the idea of a disposable razor blade.

1903 Gillette and his partner, inventor William Nickerson, open for business above a Boston fish market.

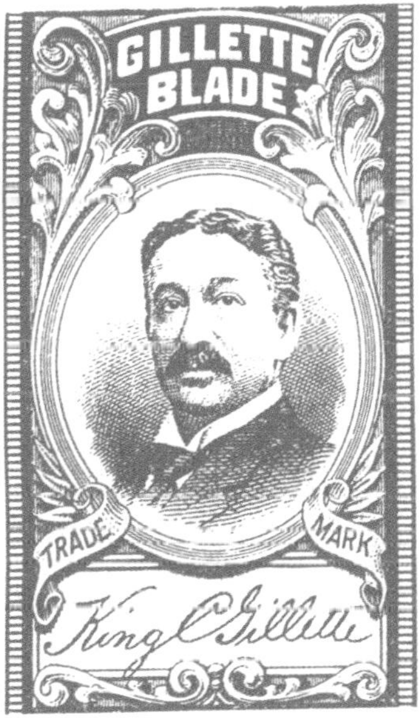

1906 Arnold Fountain Safety Razor Company produces the first pen-shaped razor—perfect for the traveling businessman.

1910 Willis G. Shockey obtains a patent for the first windup safety razor, the precursor of the electric shaver.

1917 The U.S. Congress declares war on Germany and the American government orders 3.5 million razors and 36 million blades for its armed forces. Proper hygiene in the appalling conditions of trench warfare is not the military command's only concern; a man gets a tighter seal on his gas mask if he is clean-shaven. (British soldiers are issued straight razors, the military only converting to the safety razor in 1920.)

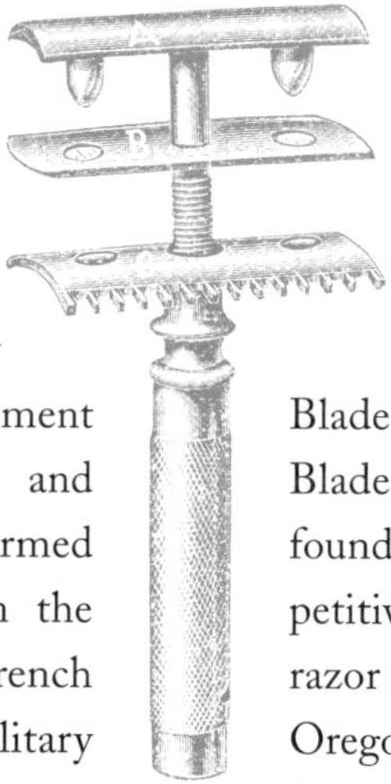

Above: Gillette safety razor circa 1905

1931 Lt. Col. Jacob Schick begins to market an electric dry shaver that works on oscillating clippers.

1932 The Gillette Company begins manufacturing its Blue Blade (followed by the Thin Blade in 1938); the company founder dies; and despite competitive pricing of disposable razor blades, lumberjacks in Oregon are reported to be giving each other perfect shaves with honed axes.

1935 Aqua Velva is introduced.

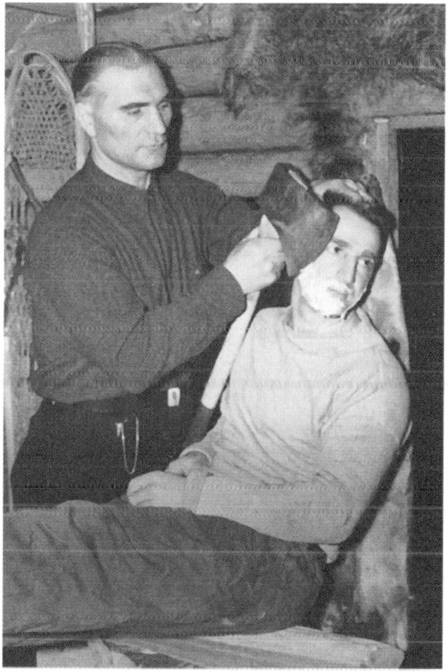

Above: Shaving with axes was a common practice in the North Woods. Here, world-champion wood chopper Perry Greene gives Eber Peck a shave.

1938 Old Spice hits the market and is, to this day, the best-selling brand in the country—smells like Dad.

1939 Gillette sponsors its first World Series between the New York Yankees and the Cincinnati Reds, and begins broadcasting the *Cavalcade of Sports*, bringing baseball, football, horse racing, and boxing into the homes of American sports fans.

1949 English Leather appears.

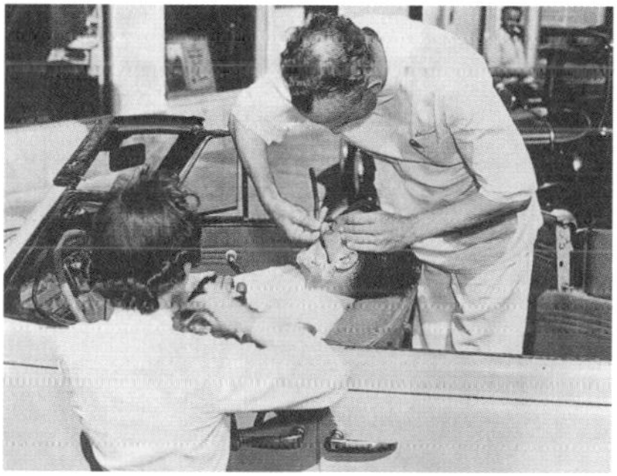

Above: After VJ Day, Americans could order a burger and fries or watch a movie without ever leaving their cars. In Miami, a guy could get a shave and a manicure as well.

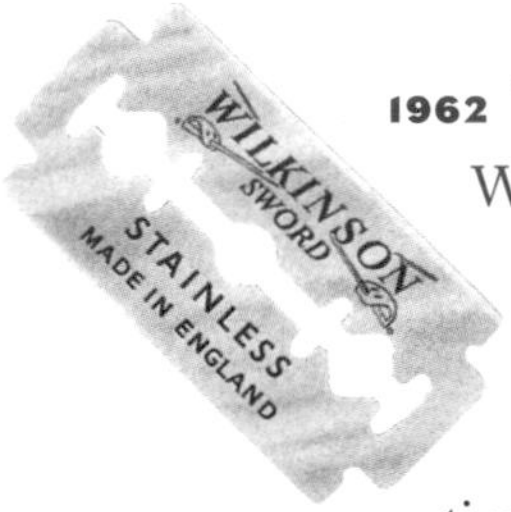

1962 The small British firm Wilkinson Sword, Ltd., markets its new Super Sword-Edge blade, which lasts five times longer than any other brand. American Safety Razor, Schick, and Gillette soon follow suit with stainless steel blades of their own.

1964 Brut aftershave emerges—what your older brother wears on dates in high school.

Below: In 1969, John Lennon and Yoko Ono traveled the world staging their "bed-in for peace."

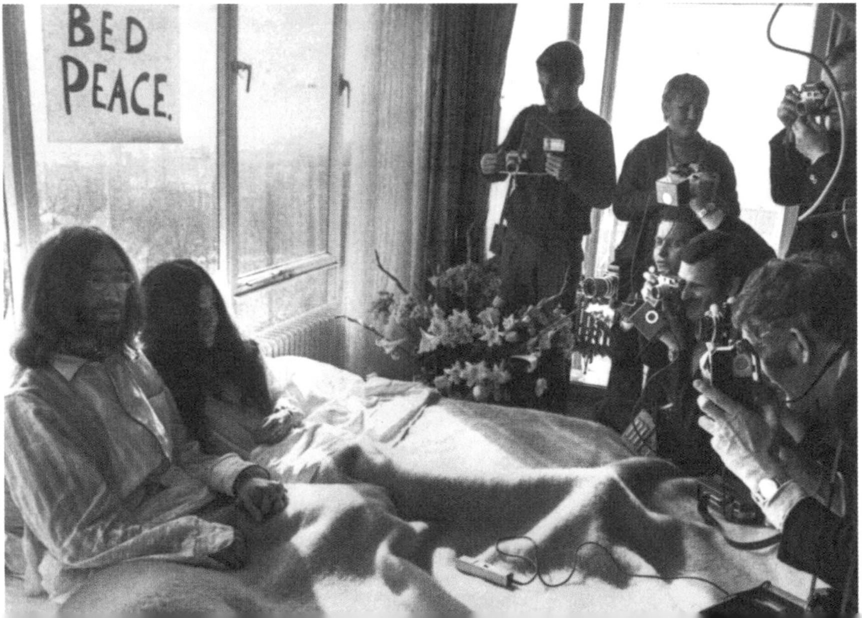

1965 First cartridge razor appears. Each cartridge contains a blade and is inserted in a plastic razor handle. (The idea originated in the 1930s.)

Late 1960s Barbers want for work as hippies and youth protesting American involvement in Vietnam grow their hair long in opposition to the Establishment.

1971 Gillette introduces the Trac II (Trac stands for "twin blade razor and cartridge"). Six years later the Atra razor (which originally stood for "Australian Test Razor" before it became "automatic tracking razor action") is introduced. It features a twin-bladed cartridge on a pivot that adjusts to the contours of the face, keeping the blades at the best cutting angle.

1972 French industrialist Marcel Bich invents the first cheap plastic disposable razor with the blade built into the head.

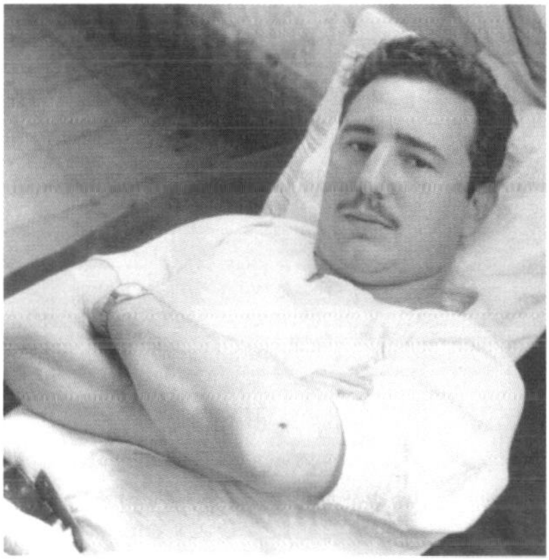

Above: Fidel Castro, 1957

1977 Fidel Castro tells Barbara Walters the reason he grew his beard during his guerrilla period in the Sierra Maestra is that his supply of Gillette blades had been cut off;

eight years later, he tells a television reporter in Rio de Janeiro that by not shaving his beard he saves up to ten days per year, time he can use for his various revolutionary activities.

Below: May 11, 1995. One man shaves another to demonstrate the mechanical hands of a remote handling device to be used in nuclear research.

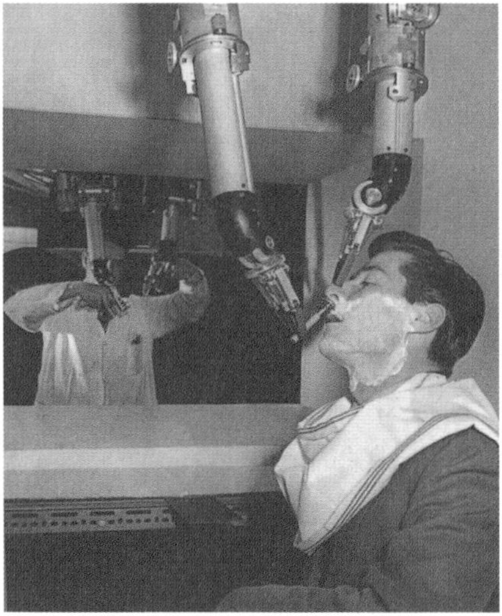

1979 The Schick plant closes and Norelco takes over the manufacturing and trademark rights.

1991 Gillette's best-selling razor ever, the Sensor Excel with a pivoting head, double blade, and lubricating strip, hits the market.

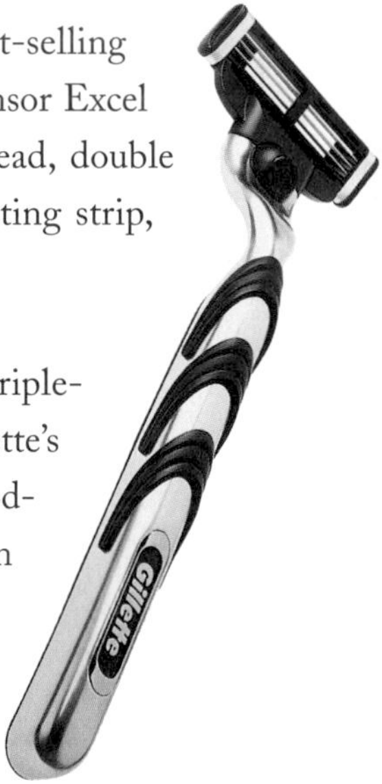

1998 The first triple-bladed razor, Gillette's Mach 3, is the product of $750 million in manufacturing and development costs.

Right: Former New York Knick Anthony Mason shaves phrases such as "Back to D" and "It's in God's Hands" into his hair.

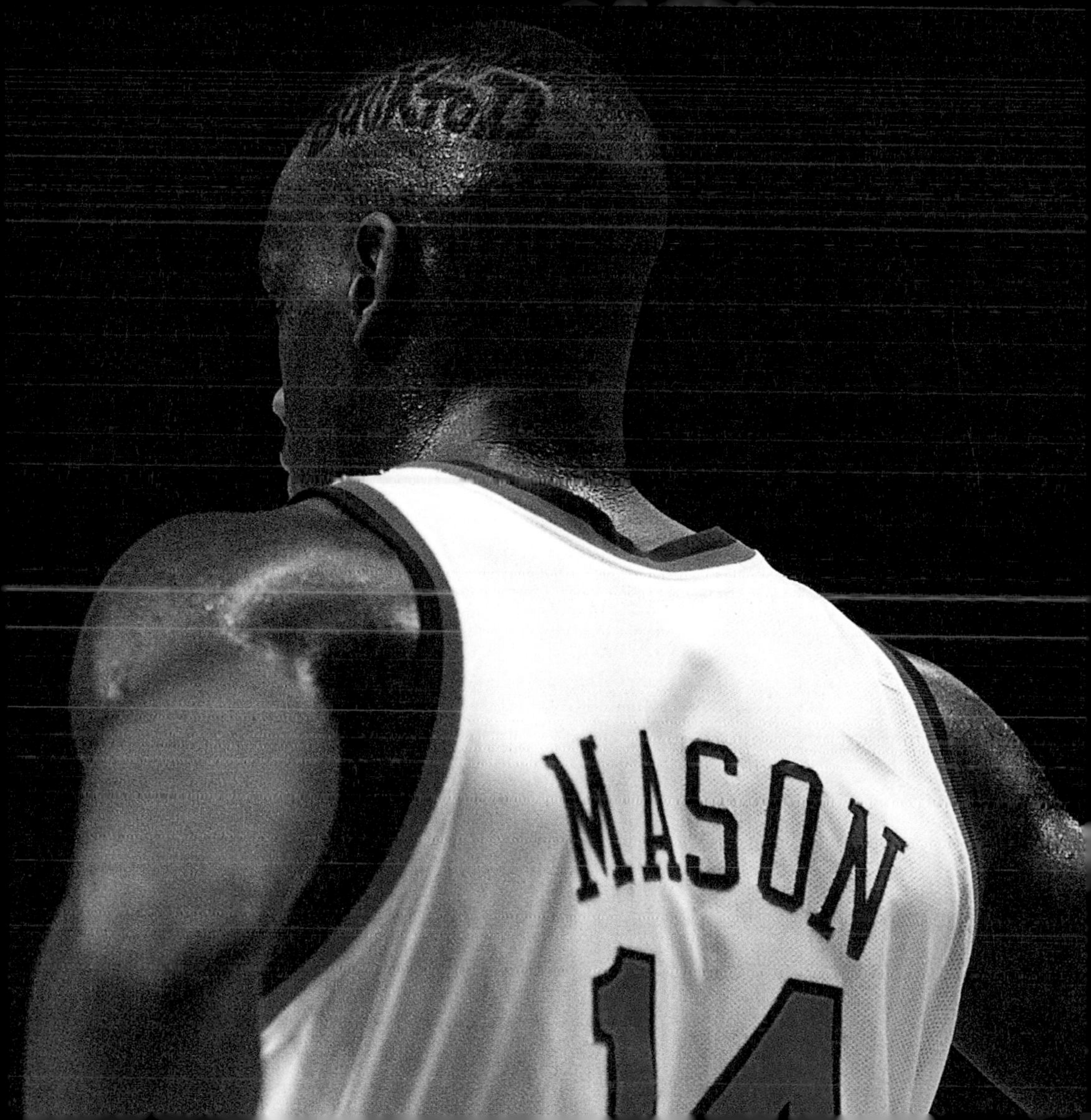
MASON
14

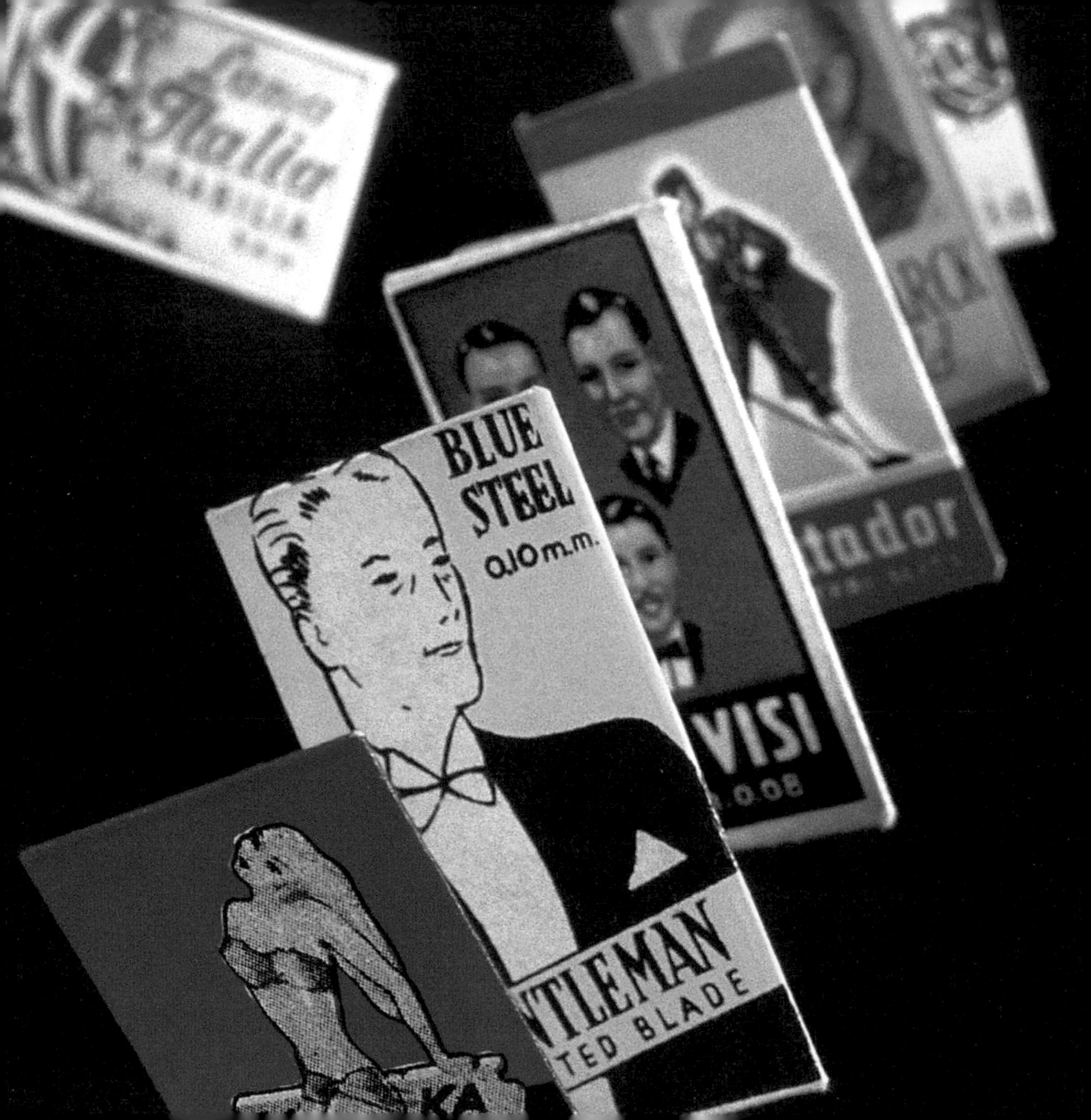
BLUE STEEL
0,10 m.m.
NTLEMAN
TED BLADE
VISI
tador

SNAIL DARTERS

As students of geology know, the earth's layers are littered with failed evolutionary experiments, the fossils of creatures whose attempts to be fruitful and multiply were unsuccessful, leaving their petrified remains for us to puzzle over. So, too, with shaving. Razor blade companies have produced quite a number of dinosaurs, dodos, and snail darters over the years. Some never found favor with the shaving public, some found favor but not forever. The inner sheathing of bathroom medicine cabinets, the discarded carriages of Pullman sleeping cars, and the lower levels of old municipal landfills are stuffed with discarded blades. Some people even collect them, but these few dedicated souls are not enough to save the names of extinct brands from oblivion.

THE ACME
MUSTACHE GUARD.
Solid Comfort while Eating.
No Use for Napkins.
Neat and simple, easily and quickly adjusted. Does not interfere with free use of mouth.
WORKS PERFECTLY.
Made of gold and silver plate. Can be carried in vest pocket. Every genteel person should have one. Two sizes, large and medium. Mention size when ordering. Price $1.00. Sent by mail to any address. Sold only by the
Acme Novelty Co.,
Omaha, Neb.

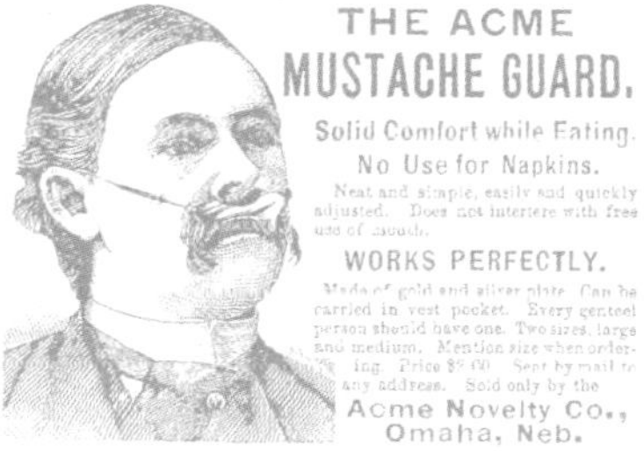

Here then is a memorial list of the names of some of those dead brands:

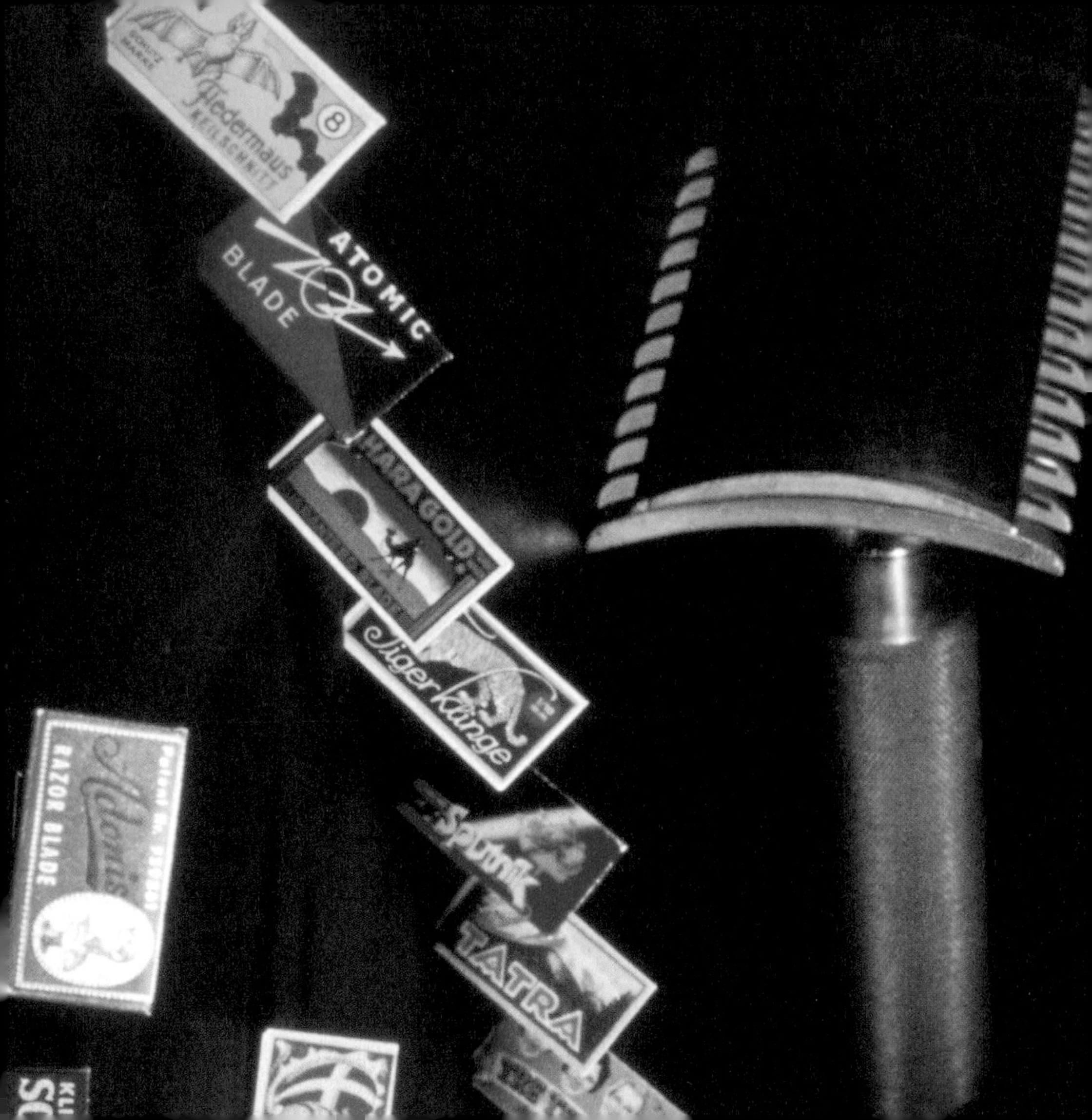
Fledermaus
KEILSCHNITT
ATOMIC
BLADE
Tiger Klinge
Sputnik
TATRA
Adonis
RAZOR BLADE

Acme, Acorn, Adams, Admiral, Adoration, Aktlebolaget, Alert, All-in-One, Alpine, Alwin, Any-Angle, Apollo, Aquapruf, Aristocrat, Arkeen, Autocrat, Avoid 5 O'Clock Shadow, Babe Ruth, Ball, Bantam, Barbarossa, Barber's Friend, Barber's Own, Barber's Pet, Barber's Quartet, B-B, Ben Hur, Big Ben, Big Boy Blue, Big Chief, Big Fellow, Big Stick, Big Wheel, Black Demon, Black Foot, Black Tank, the Blacky, Brisk, Brownie, Buddy, Budget, Buffalo, Bulls Eye, B-Y, Cameo, Campus, Carnival, Casco, Casino, Cell-o Thin, Centennial, Century of Progress, Chairman, Charm, Chase, Cheerio, Chef au Ritz, Chippendale, Chum, Clix, Clover, Club, Congress, Conqueror, Copper King, Corn Husker, Cosmo, Country Club, Credo, Croce di Malta, Czar of Russia, Daily, Daisy, Damascus, Dandy, Demon Spark, Diana, Diplomat, Dixie, Doll, Don Juan, Dragon, Dubl-Duck, Eclipse, Eldorado, Empire Eskimo, Esquire, Everybody's, Excalibur, Excello, E-Z-Flo, EZ Shave, Falcon, Fashionable, Fax, Flash, Float-Blade, Fortune, Four Hundred, Friendly, Full Dress, GAY, Gazelle, Gem, Gilt Edge, Gold Medal, Gold'n Honey, Gold Nugget, Gold Tone, Good Humor, Good Luck, Good Value, Grand Prize, Holiday, Hollywood, Husky, Hustler, Ile de France, Imco, Imperial, Indicator, Jai Alai, Jet, Jewel, Jockey, Jupiter, Jury, Kant-Rust, Katz, Ked, Keen Kutter, Keg, King of Shaves, Kooledge, Lido, Lightning, Lucky Boy, Lucky Stroke, Mac, Magmatic, Major, Maple, Mariposa, Master Action, Metropolitan, Micromatic, Midget, Mike, Milord, Minora, Mystery Edge, My-Te-Fine, Nat, Navy Blue, Nobby, Nox-All, Okey, Once, Opera, Optimus, Over, Owl, Pal, Palm, Palmolive, Paragon, Paramount, Pard, Parex, Peerless, Penguin, Peoples, Perfect, Permedge, Phantom, Pilot, Pontiac, Presto, Prime, Prince, Professor, Pronto, Protex, Pullman, Purple, Radio, Rajah, Ravin,

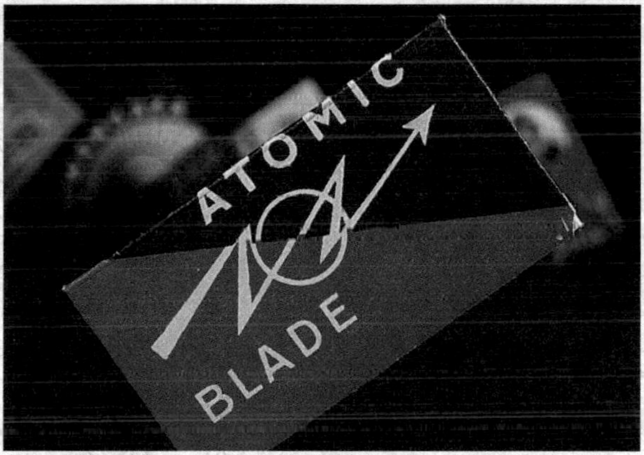

Ray-Steel, Razolite, Red Cap, Red Circle, Red Devil, Regatta, Revelation, Reversible, Rex, Ring Thin, Rio, Ritz, Rodeo, Salambo, Samson, Sanitax, Sapphire, Sarita , Sav-A-Blade, Savage, Scotch 40 Day, Scotty, Sentinel, Sentry, Shamrock, Sharps in Flats, Shav-a-way, Sha-Ve-Zee, Shav-O, Shav-Rite, Shav-Ur-Self, Shawmut, Sheffield, Shelby, Shield, Silver King, Silver Star, Simplex, Sir, Sir Henry, Sir John, Sir Richard, Sir Roger, Sisters, Six O'Clock, Smooth-Shave, Society, Solo, Span, Speed, Sportsman, Steel Town, Stetson, Swan, Swank, Sweco, Swift, Swing, Symphony, Tally Ho, Tek, Templar, Texide, Thinere, Thin-Flex, Thin-Jim, Tick Tock, Token, Top Hat, Top Notch, Tornado, Town Talk, Travalong, Trial King, Tropical, True Romance, True Story, Tuxedo, Twenty Grand, Two Bucks, Uneeda, Upat, Valley Forge, Vampire, Vellum, Whippet, White Horse, Whiz-Pak, Wil Kut, World's Fair, Wright, Wrigley, Yale, Zinn.

Amen.

George Babbitt Makes His Morning Toilette

The bath-mat was wrinkled and the floor was wet. . . . He slipped on the mat, and slid against the tub. He said, "Damn!" Furiously he snatched up his tube of shaving-cream, furiously he lathered, with a belligerent slapping of the unctuous brush, furiously he raked his plump cheeks with a safety-razor. It pulled. The blade was dull. He said, "Damn—oh—oh—damn it!"

He hunted through the medicine-cabinet for a packet of new razor blades (reflecting, as invariably, "Be cheaper to buy one of those dinguses and strop your own blades,") and when he discovered the packet, behind the round box of bicarbonate of soda, he thought ill of his wife for putting it there and very well of himself for not saying "Damn." But he did say it, immediately afterward, when with wet and soap-slippery fingers he tried to remove the horrible little envelope and crisp clinging oiled paper from the new blade.

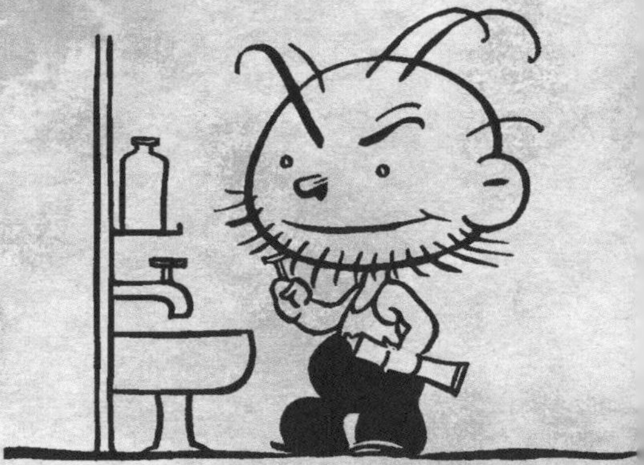

Then there was the problem, oft-pondered, never solved, of what to do with the old blade, which might imperil the fingers of his young. As usual, he tossed it on top of the medicine-cabinet, with a mental note that some day he must remove the fifty or sixty other blades that were also temporarily piled up there. He finished his shaving in a growing testiness increased by his spinning headache and by the emptiness in his stomach. When he was done, his round face smooth and steamy and his eyes stinging from soapy water, he reached for a towel. . . .

Sinclair Lewis, *Babbitt*

King Camp Gillette
(1855–1932)

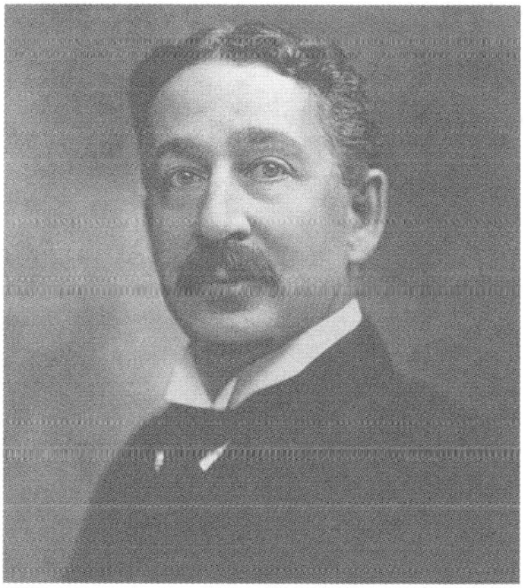

"On one particular morning when I started to shave, I found my razor dull, and it was not only dull, but it was beyond the point of successful stropping. It needed honing, too, for which it must be taken to a barber or to a cutler. As I stood there with the razor in my hand, my eye resting on it as lightly as a bird settling down on its nest, the Gillette razor was born."

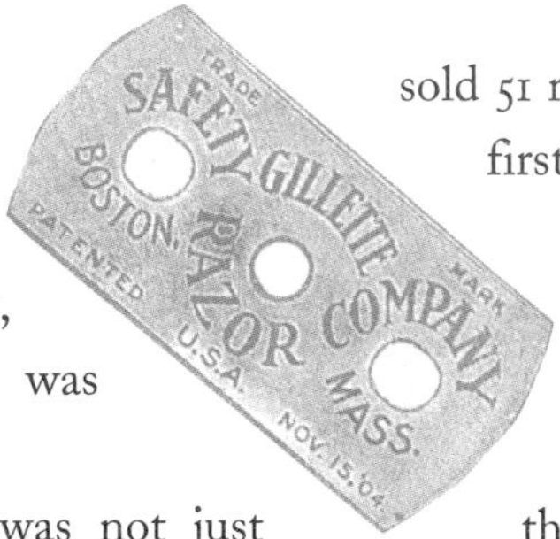

Gillette's genius was not just the invention of two cutting edges rather than one, but the idea that once the blade no longer did the job, it should be discarded. His safety razor is the perfect exemplar of disposability, the modern commercial principle that requires that a given product perform well but that it deteriorate rapidly. If a product is to be a success and survive, it must be imperfect.

King Camp Gillette and his partner, William Nickerson, opened for business in 1903. They sold 51 razors and 168 blades the first year; 90,000 razors and 2.4 million blades the next year; and by 1905, they were up to 250,000 sets. Clearly, the safety razor answered a need.

But World War I was really the making of the Gillette Company: American troops were issued Gillette shaving kits rather than straight razors and millions of men who, in the normal course of things, would have sought out a barber, learned to shave themselves unaided. After the Armistice, these young men constituted a vast contingent of new customers,

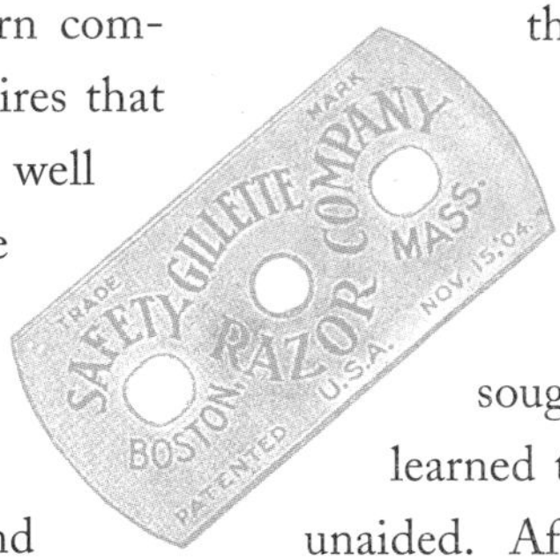

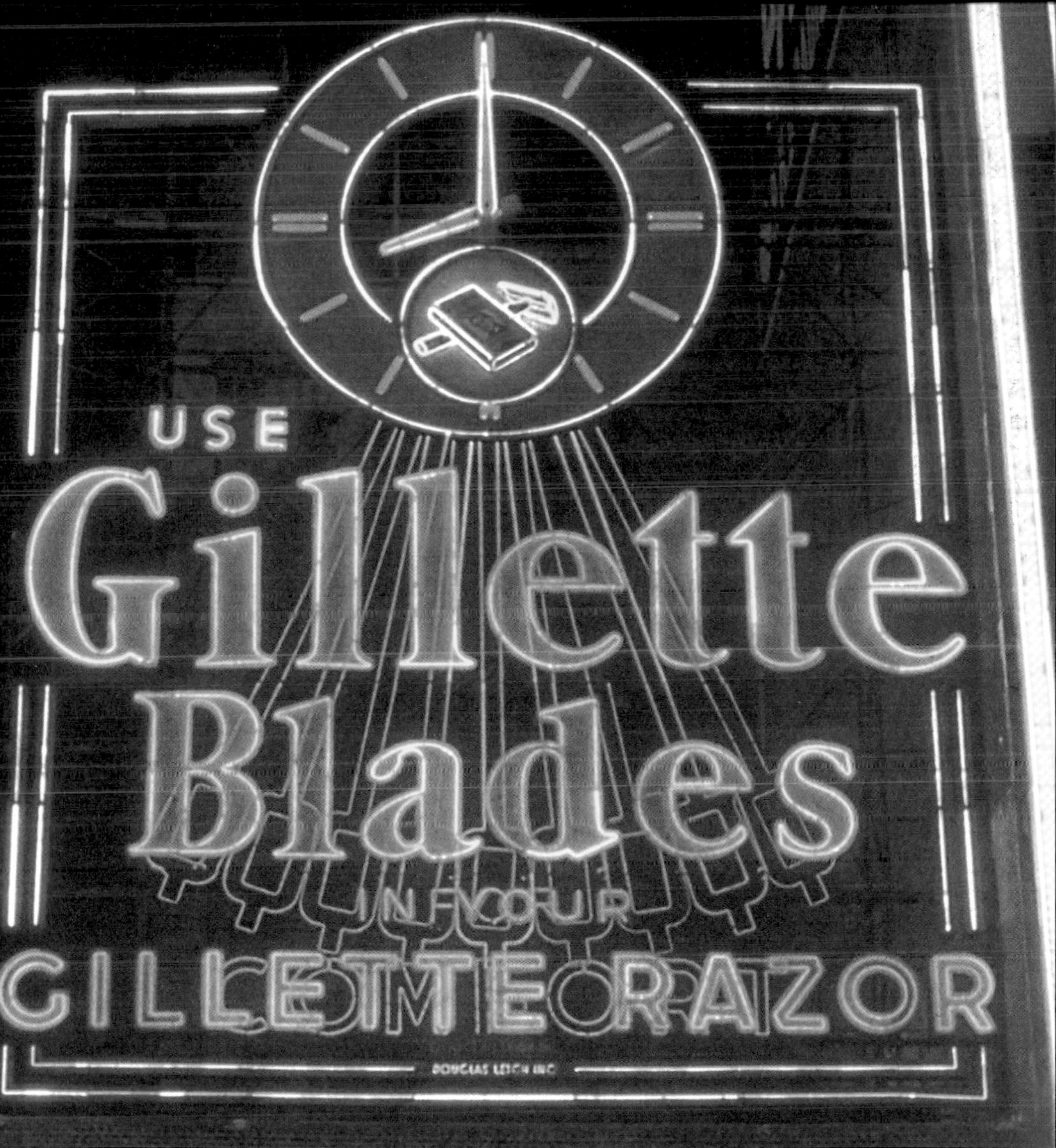
USE
Gillette
Blades
IN YOUR
GILLETTE RAZOR
DOUGLAS LEIGH INC

ready to buy blades to fit the safety razors they had learned to use in the military.

For years after his death, King Camp Gillette still had the most familiar face humanity had ever known. Almost from the beginning of his company, his face and signature appeared on every single razor blade wrapping the company produced. The portrait of a youngish man, smooth-chinned but with a luxuriant mustache, was reproduced more often than that of Jesus Christ, Mickey Mouse, or the Buddha. In villages off the edge of the map, where neither the lettering on the package nor his signature meant anything, local people still knew enough to ask for "man-face" brand blades.

Colonel Jacob Schick
(1878–1937)

Ever since electricity became available at the turn of the century, inventors had been trying to apply it to shaving. But it was Lt. Col. Jacob Schick who fathered the invention in 1931. His inspiration came to him as he recuperated from a sprained ankle in an Alaskan gold-mining camp in 1910. The forty-degree-below-zero weather made shaving difficult, and he began thinking there must be a better way.

Thirteen years later, Schick obtained his first patent, for a large, hand-held, universal motor with a remote cutting head; the motor was held in one hand, the cutting head in the other. He'd been thinking about it for a decade, but he had to

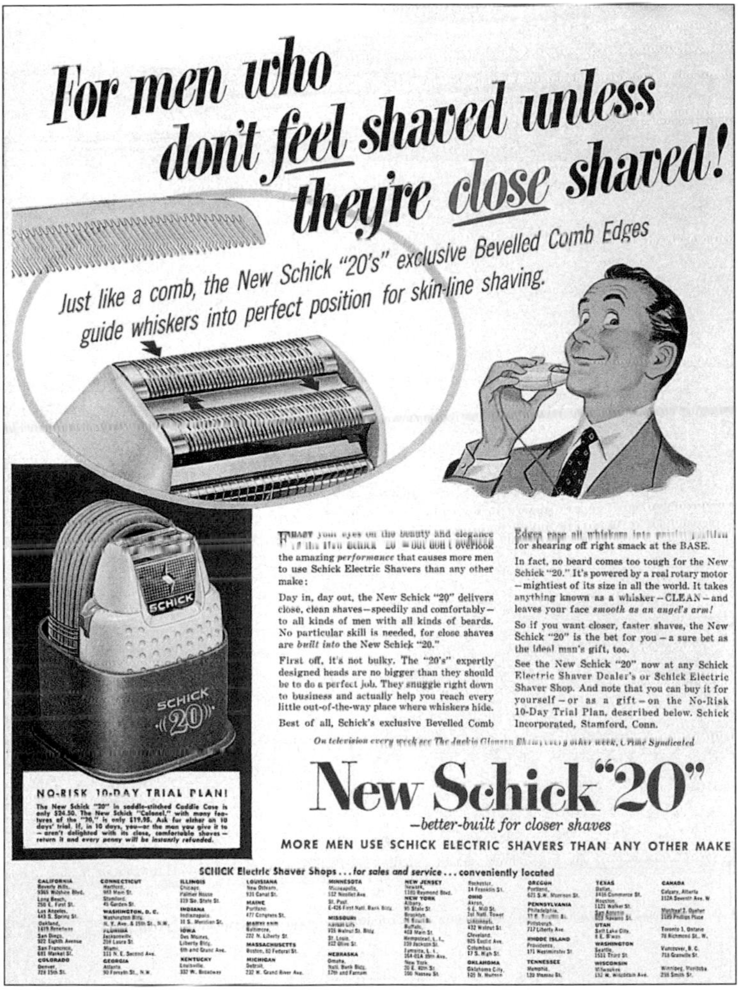
For men who don't feel shaved unless they're close shaved!
Just like a comb, the New Schick "20's" exclusive Bevelled Comb Edges guide whiskers into perfect position for skin-line shaving.
SCHICK
SCHICK 20
the amazing performance that causes more men to use Schick Electric Shavers than any other make:
Day in, day out, the New Schick "20" delivers close, clean shaves—speedily and comfortably—to all kinds of men with all kinds of beards. No particular skill is needed, for close shaves are built into the New Schick "20."
First off, it's not bulky. The "20's" expertly designed heads are no bigger than they should be to do a perfect job. They snuggle right down to business and actually help you reach every little out-of-the-way place where whiskers hide.
Best of all, Schick's exclusive Bevelled Comb
for shearing off right smack at the BASE.
In fact, no beard comes too tough for the New Schick "20." It's powered by a real rotary motor—mightiest of its size in all the world. It takes anything known as a whisker—CLEAN—and leaves your face smooth as an angel's arm!
So if you want closer, faster shaves, the New Schick "20" is the bet for you—a sure bet as the ideal man's gift, too.
See the New Schick "20" now at any Schick Electric Shaver Dealer's or Schick Electric Shaver Shop. And note that you can buy it for yourself—or as a gift—on the No-Risk 10-Day Trial Plan, described below. Schick Incorporated, Stamford, Conn.
NO-RISK 10-DAY TRIAL PLAN!
The New Schick "20" in saddle-stitched Caddie Case is only $24.50. The New Schick "Colonel," with many features of the "20," is only $19.95. Ask for either on 10 days' trial. If, in 10 days, you—or the man you give it to—aren't delighted with its close, comfortable shaves—return it and every penny will be instantly refunded.
New Schick "20"
—better-built for closer shaves
MORE MEN USE SCHICK ELECTRIC SHAVERS THAN ANY OTHER MAKE
SCHICK Electric Shaver Shops . . . for sales and service . . . conveniently located

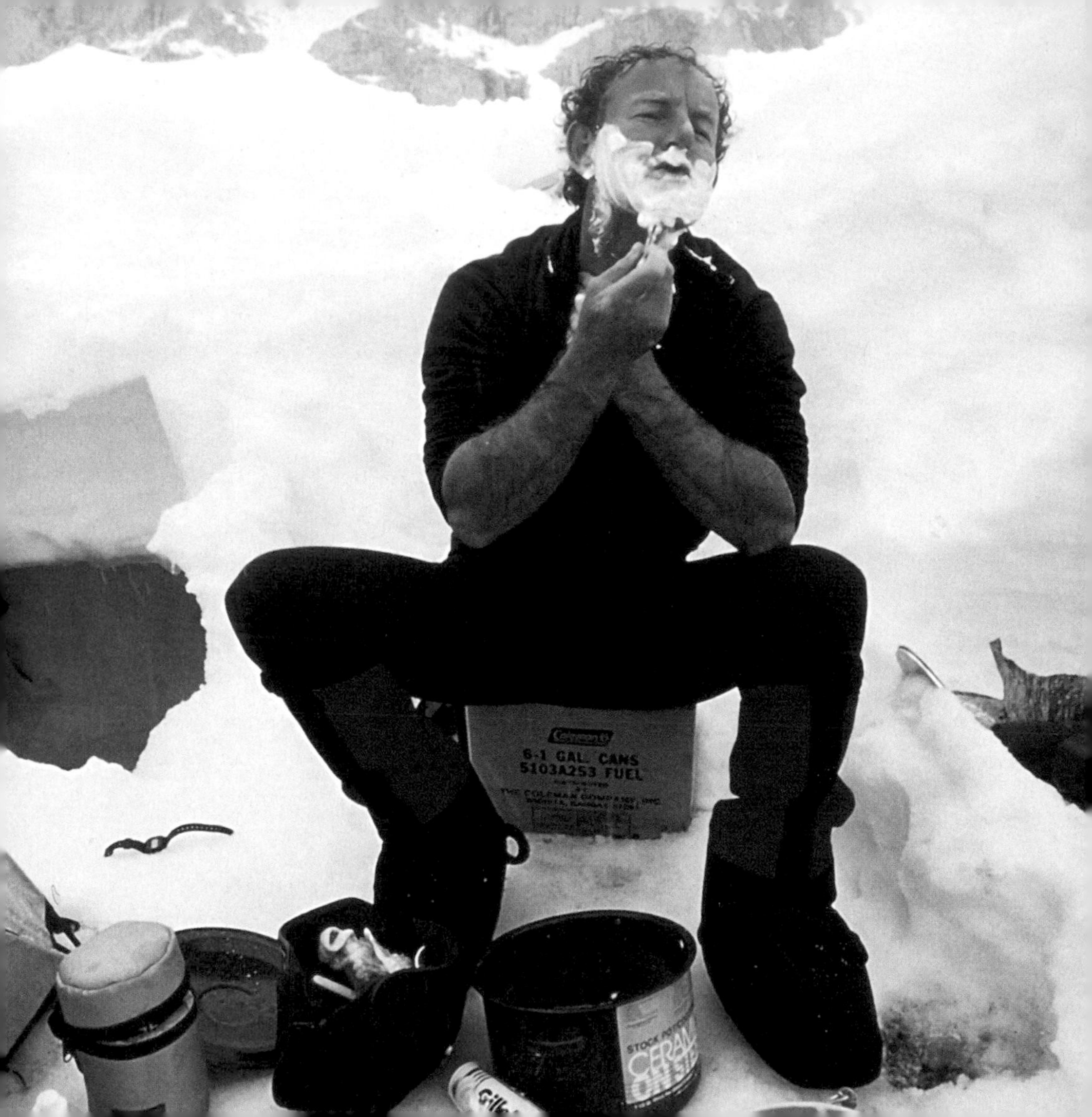
6-1 GAL. CANS
5103A253 FUEL

wait until technology caught up with his idea. A true electric shaver couldn't be developed until electric motors got small enough to be housed in hand-held appliances. This came about in the 1920s, simultaneously with the electrification of more and more households.

In the meantime, Schick placed the Magazine Repeating Razor on the market in 1926. Touted as "one of the greatest mechanical inventions of the twentieth century," it was a wet razor that stored twenty blades in its handle and, by operation of a handle plunger, ejected a dull blade and installed a new one. Consumers were now protected from handling the dangerous blades.

Schick sold the company a year later to get capital for the manufacture and marketing of his dry shaver. The first one sold for $25 in 1931 and represented a considerable advance over his original idea. It was smaller and more powerful; now, an oscillating induction motor—for its size, the most powerful in the world—drove a sliding cutter inside a slotted shearing head, all housed in a smooth, black Bakelite shell. Public acceptance was underwhelming; the Depression was not the best time for an expensive new product to take off, but his dry shaver survived and inspired others.

Left: Even in an Alaskan snowfield, a man with the right attitude and the right equipment can look his best.

Which Razor Is Best?

Tastes differ. The razor one man swears by, another abjures. However, it's not merely a matter of taste. Twin blades do work better than single ones. Hysteresis is the reason: As the double-bladed razor advances, the first blade lops off each individual whisker and pulls it slightly out of its follicle. The second blade, millimeters behind the first, cuts the hair even shorter before it can retract. QED, a closer shave.

So if two blades shave closer than one, the closest possible shave would be achieved with some system of gang-mowers, right? Or at least the three-bladed wonder, Gillette's Mach 3? Not necessarily. Some men swear by it. Others find its larger head makes shaving under the nose tricky. Because it's not easy to tell at first where the new blades meet the face, trimming sideburns or a beard may require practice. On the other hand, the design lends itself to shaving large areas. So it's ideal for women's legs and body builder's backs. The verdict:

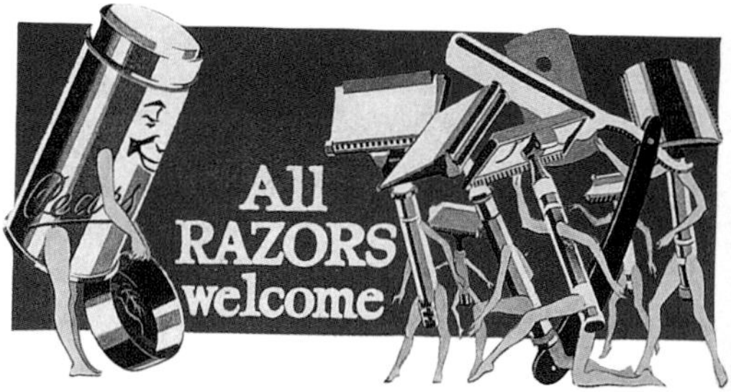

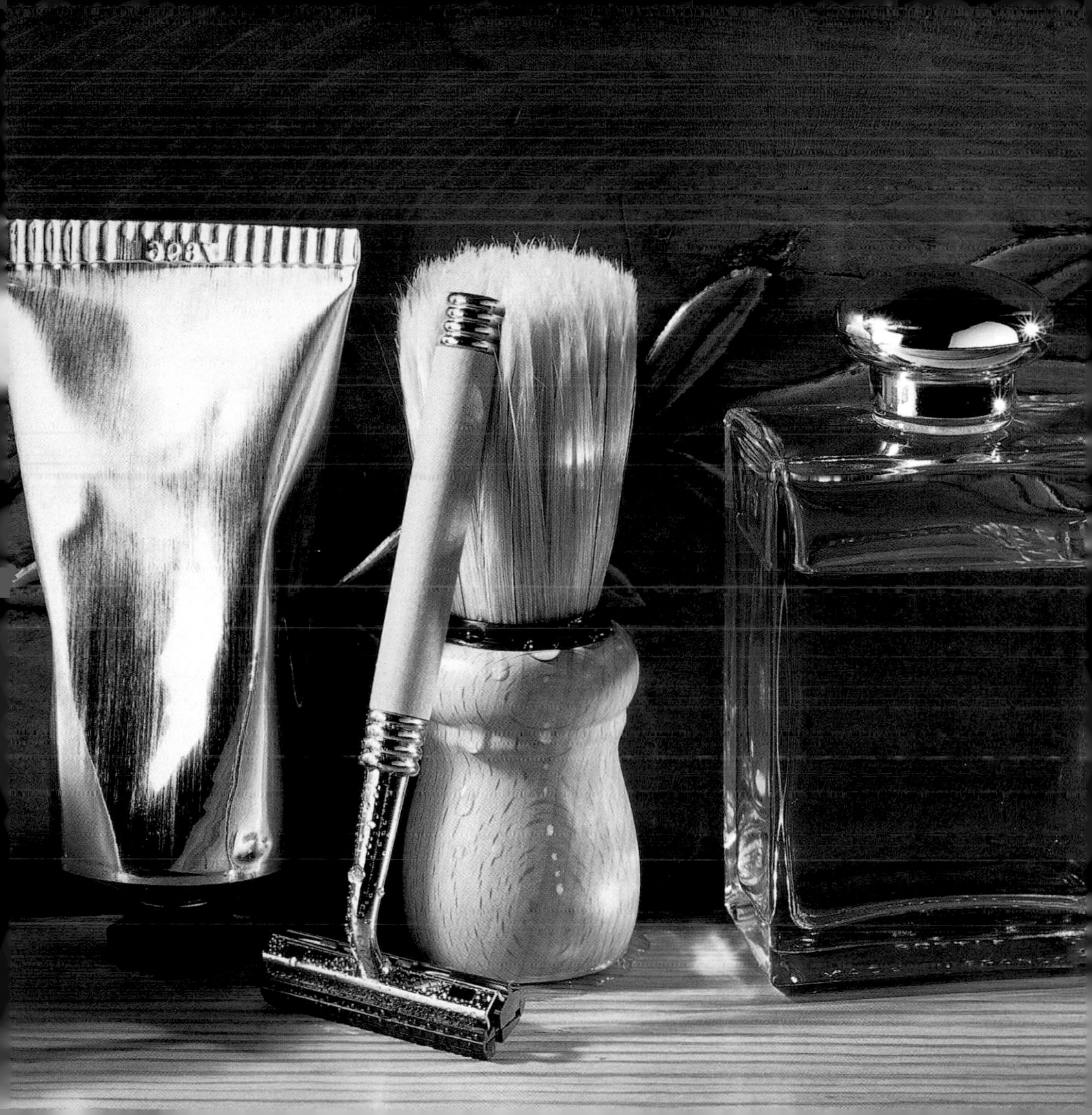

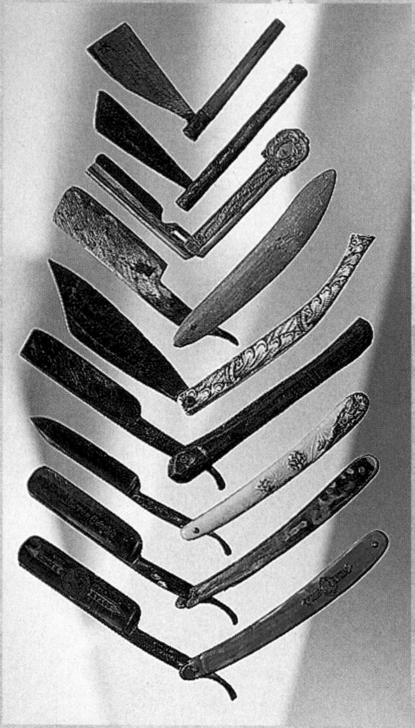

The Razor

It knows my surface
physiognomy—keen where it can
and cannot glide—better than
myself. (Will I have, when this

is done, a face I recognize,
a profile left, or right?) Morning
cuts the pattern for the adolescent owning
of the day to come. Its kiss,

thin-lipped, sends me on
to what I deem familiar
as facsimile of what we are,
and what I am—Homo erectus of one

more day of man, shorn
of beard and cave and flint,
left behind in mirror, skinned
of rudimentary Cro-Magnon and Piltdown.

Marvin Solomon

the Mach 3 is an excellent razor—but so are the newest twin blades.

Although disposable razors are more popular with the American public and cheaper, cartridge razors are easier to use and give a few more shaves than disposables. In shaving instruments, you pretty much get what you pay for.

Mirror, Mirror

A mirror has no heart
but plenty of ideas.
Malcolm de Chazal

You actually can shave without a mirror. Saunas and steam rooms, where a mirror either wouldn't work or would look foolish, are excellent places to shave; whiskers practically slide off your jaw, and a pass of your palm indicates what remains to be done.

For most other venues, however, a mirror is a plus while shaving. Let's start with the obvious: A well-lighted mirror is preferable to a dark one; a clear mirror is preferable to a steamy one; and if you like

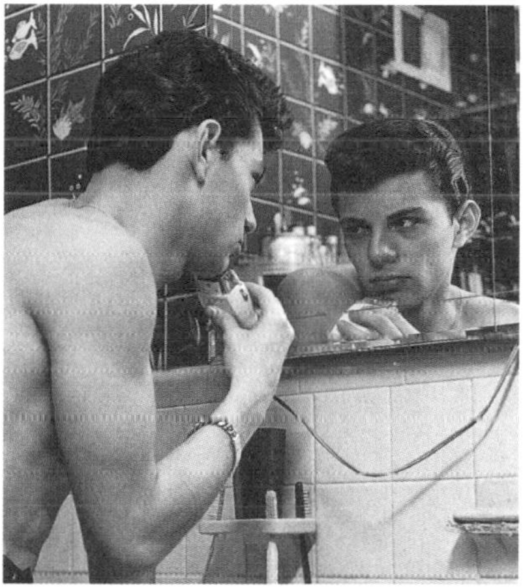

Above: Frankie Avalon demonstrates good teen idol techniques: He looks himself in the eye. And he's sincere.

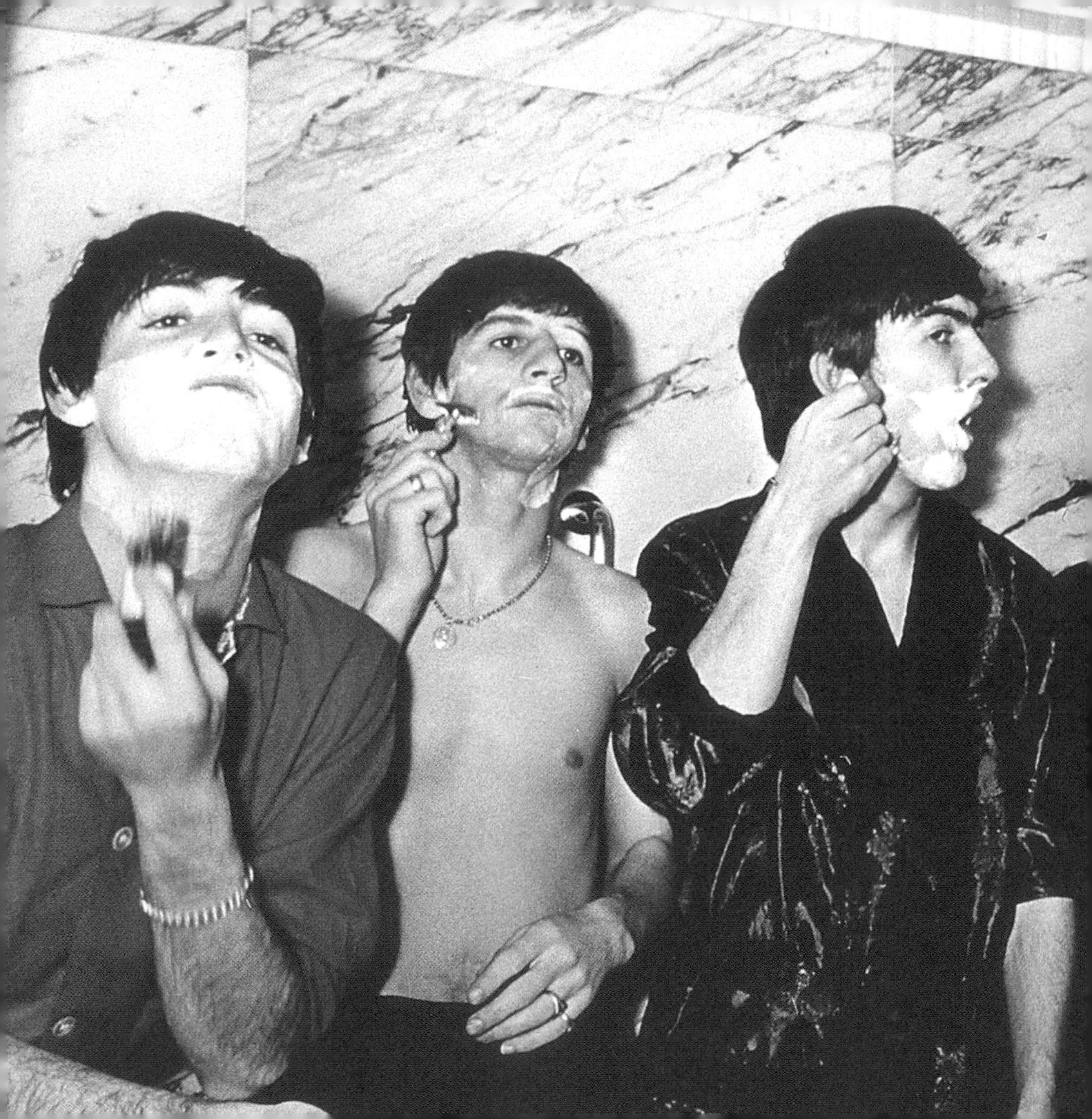

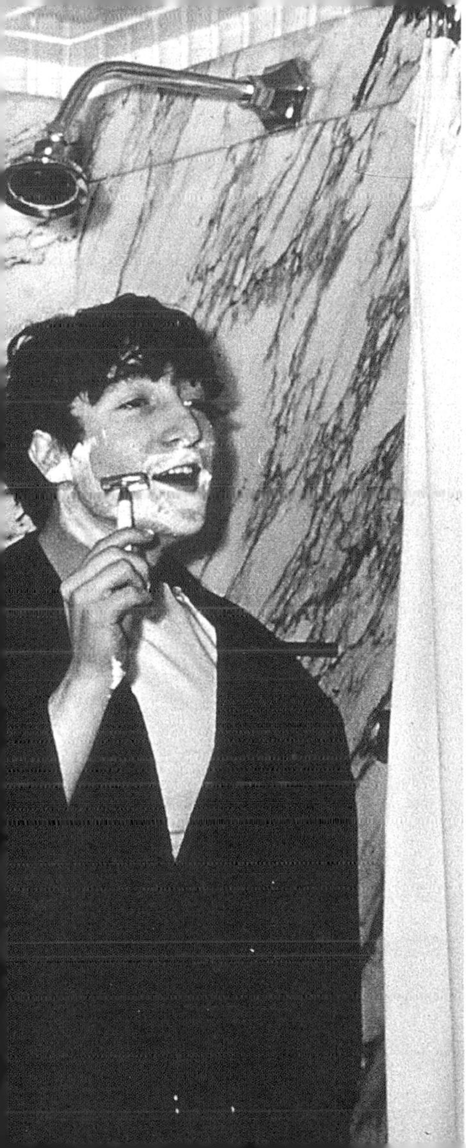

to shave in the shower and want to see yourself while you're doing it, acrylic fog-free mirrors are the way to go. Many of them attach to the showerhead and circulate hot water to the rear of the reflecting surface, thus preventing condensation.

What you don't need although you may think you do is a magnifying mirror. An ordinary man with ordinary beard growth doesn't really need to see his pores in such detail. A magnifying mirror only encourages the second big shaving mistake (cheap, dull blades are number one): shaving too close.

Face it: Even regular mirrors are scary places to visit. Unless he is one of those rare men who

Left: If "She Came in Through the Bathroom Window," it would be best to "Act Naturally" and pretend to shave.

is unselfconsciously, unabashedly interested in his own looks, a man barely sees himself in the course of the morning ablutions. Because he sees that same face, day in and day out, he is less able to observe the signs of sadness or decay or indisposition so obvious to everyone else. The mirror's narcotic effect allows him to age from fifteen to eighty without noticing any particular change. He notes how time and troubles have ravaged everyone around him, but his own decay is imperceptible.

Equally disquieting is the knowledge that the face you see in the mirror is not the one your friends see when they look your way. They see its opposite—the wen is to the left of your nose, not the right; the cocked eyebrow is above your right eye, not your left. If you want to know how the man your friends and relations have been greeting all your life really looks, you'll need a second mirror.

Shaving Cream, Foam, and Gel

Before there was gel, there was foam, and before there was foam there were creams, and before the creams there was plain old soap. They've all been sold to the public for well over a century; they all heal the skin, protect the pores, refresh, and restore to some degree. What has changed is not their function but the way in which they're applied. Until the middle of the eighteenth century, barbers used a sponge or the tips of their fingers—

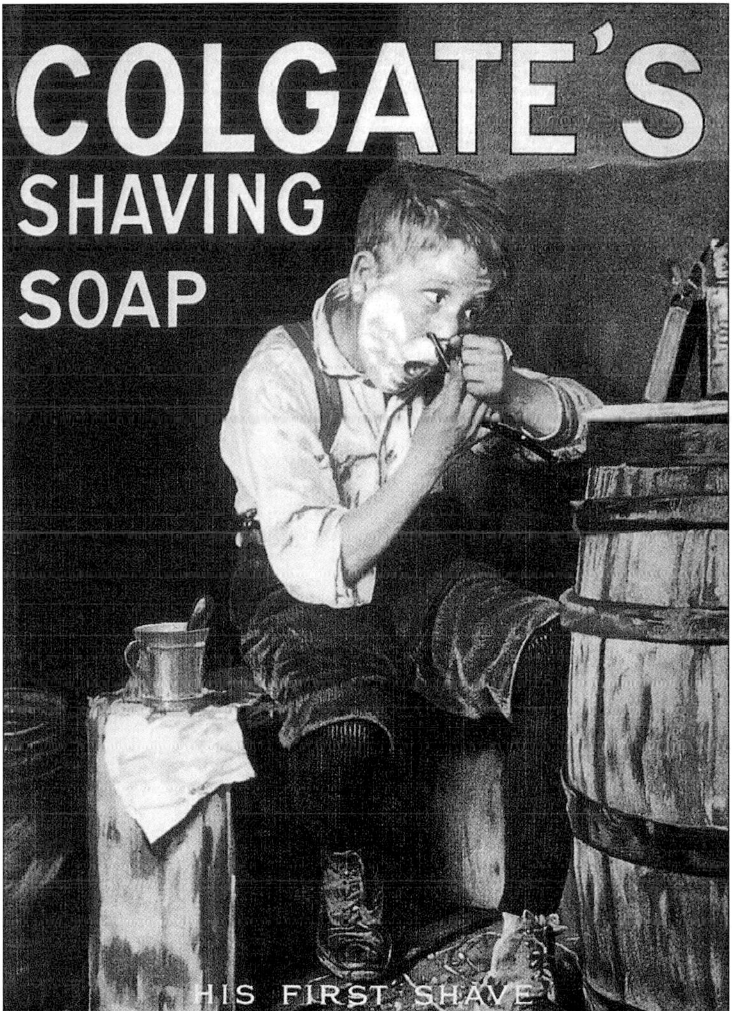

COLGATE'S
SHAVING
SOAP
HIS FIRST SHAVE

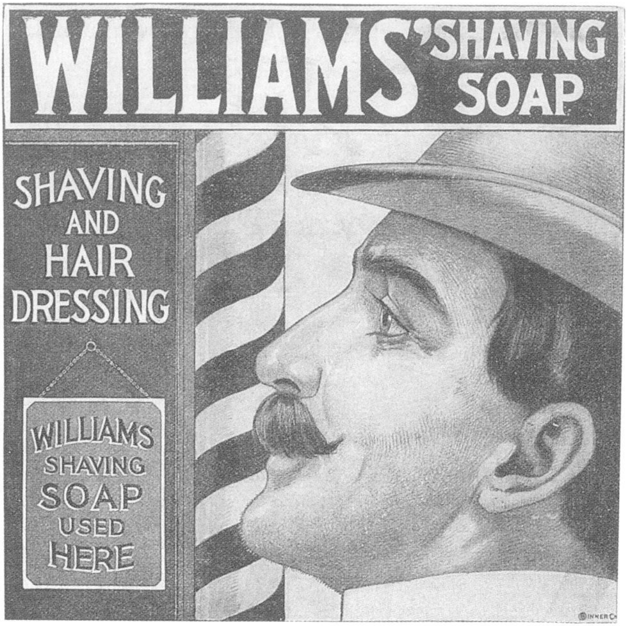

dirty fingers notwithstanding—to create a lather. (The shaving brush was introduced by the French in the 1750s, and it has held its own for nearly two centuries.)

Brushless creams were on the market by the time of the First World War. Shaving cream that came in a tube was far more convenient for the man in a hurry than a shaving brush, mug, and soap. But old habits die hard: Travel kits were available where brush and straight razor fit neatly into a brushed aluminum tube. Shaving brushes still have their aficionados

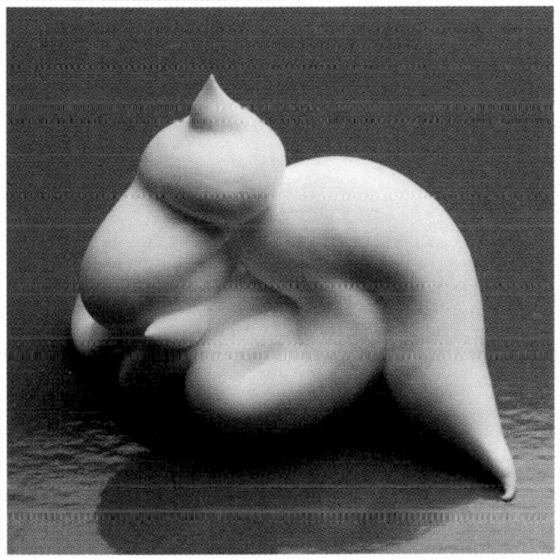

Colleges have reputations to uphold and out-of-hand fun is one of their building blocks. Rice University has the Baker 13, comprising several dozen undergraduates wearing nothing but shaving cream. The mission of Baker 13 is for each person to leave as many body prints as a twelve-ounce can of lemon-lime with aloe foam will allow. On Halloween 1992, one enthusiastic freshman attempted to leave the imprint of his buttocks on the doors of the university library. An athletic young man, his backward jump shattered the glass, and he ended up having his buttocks stitched back together in the ER. Since he hadn't had the foresight to take out liability insurance on his posterior, funds for the repair of the door were raised by selling "Save John's Ass" T-shirts.

today, but when convenience and comfort have a race, convenience usually wins.

In 1941 American chemists developed the aerosol can, a new way for dispensing insecticides. Shaving cream soon found its way into this novel container and became shaving foam. Gels, introduced fifty years later, are simply a two-times-as-slippery variation on foam. They're concentrated, semitranslucent, and they turn to lather when rubbed into the skin.

Shaving Brushes

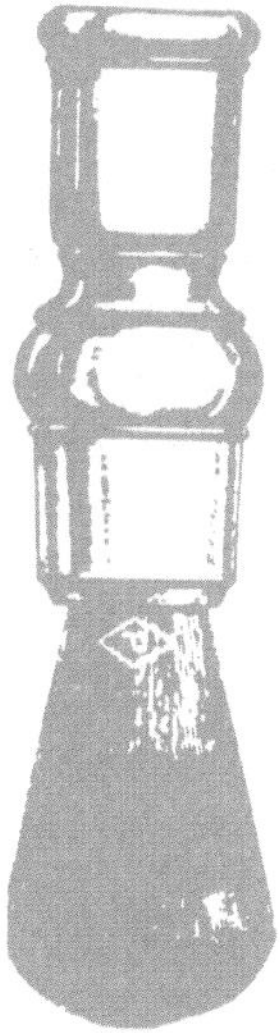

Although shaving brushes have yet to go the way of mustache crimpers and rotary hair brushes, it's been a long while since they've been the sine qua non of the morning shave.

Ordinary brushes are made of nylon or boar bristle. Really good brushes are made from a badger's stomach hair; small ones, billed as Pure Badger, start at just under $50. Even better brushes—Best Badger—use hair from the badger's back and, depending on the volume of the brush and the composition of the handle, can cost from $100 to $200. The best badger brushes are made by hand in Gloucestershire, England, by A. Simpson & Co. with the "super silver-tipped" hair from the back of the badger's neck; throw in an ivory handle, and

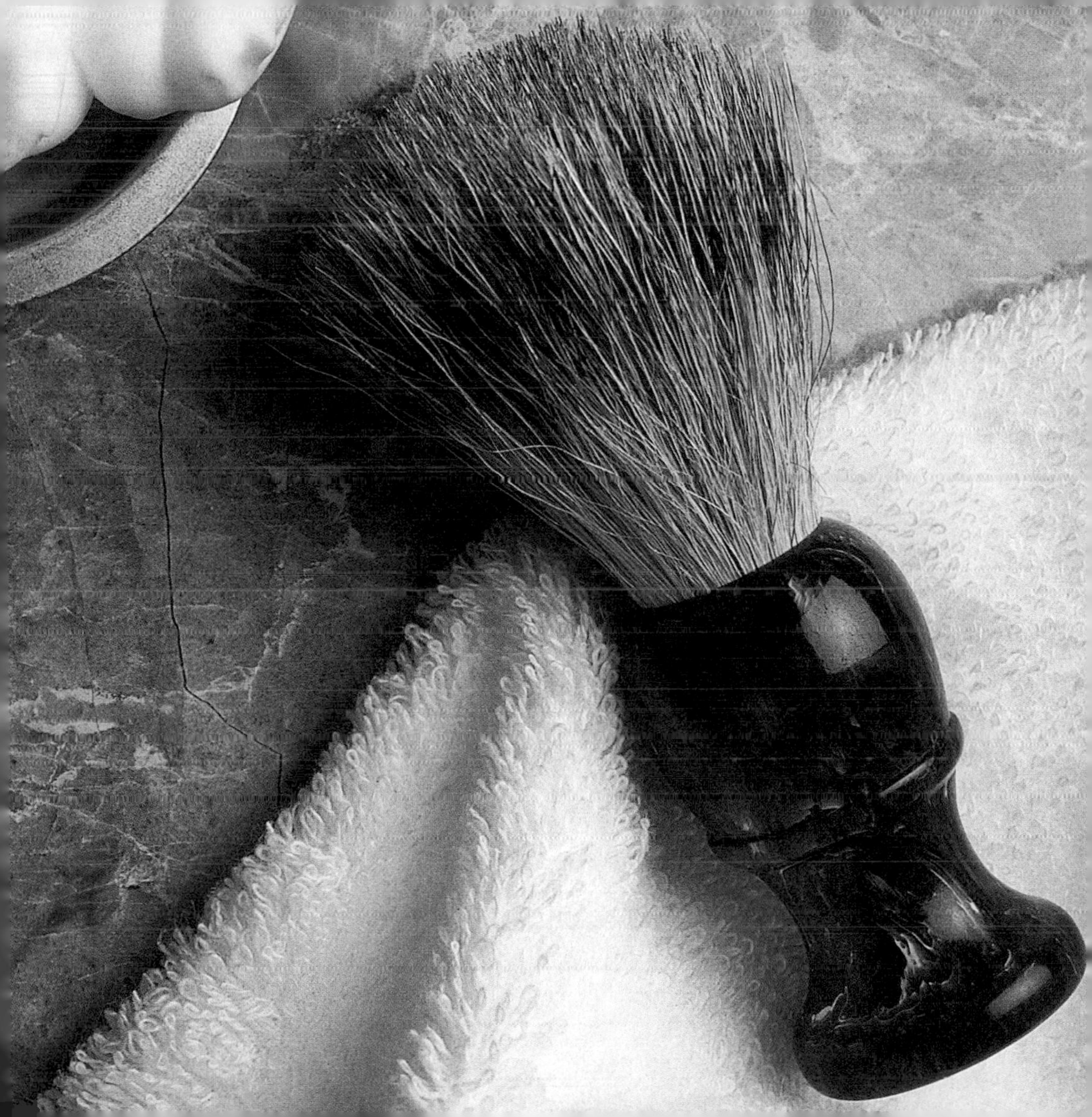

Is the eventual combined cost of all that foam, all that gel, eating away at you? You could do what lots of men do, which is just to use the bar of soap that's there on the sink. But that's a fundamentally bad idea—that soap was made for cleansing, not lubrication or rehumectification. If you don't want to spend the money on a good shaving soap, you can always make your own. Here's a recipe from *Henley's Formulas for Home and Workshop* from 1907:

Take five pounds of palm oil soap, melt it, add color if desired and incorporate the following oils: cinnamon (10 drachmas), caraway (2 drachmas), lavender (2 more drachmas), thyme (1 drachma), peppermint (45 minims), and bergamot (2 drachmas).

If you're glad we've left that can-do, inventive era well behind us but still want to try making your own shaving soap, here's a more contemporary recipe. You'll need:

½ cup clean rendered tallow
¼ cup coconut oil
1½ teaspoons melted beeswax
2 tablespoons lye flakes
½ cup cold soft water
2 tablespoons lanolin
2 tablespoons glycerine
¼ teaspoon each cloves and cinnamon

Melt together the tallow, coconut oil, and beeswax. Set aside to cool.

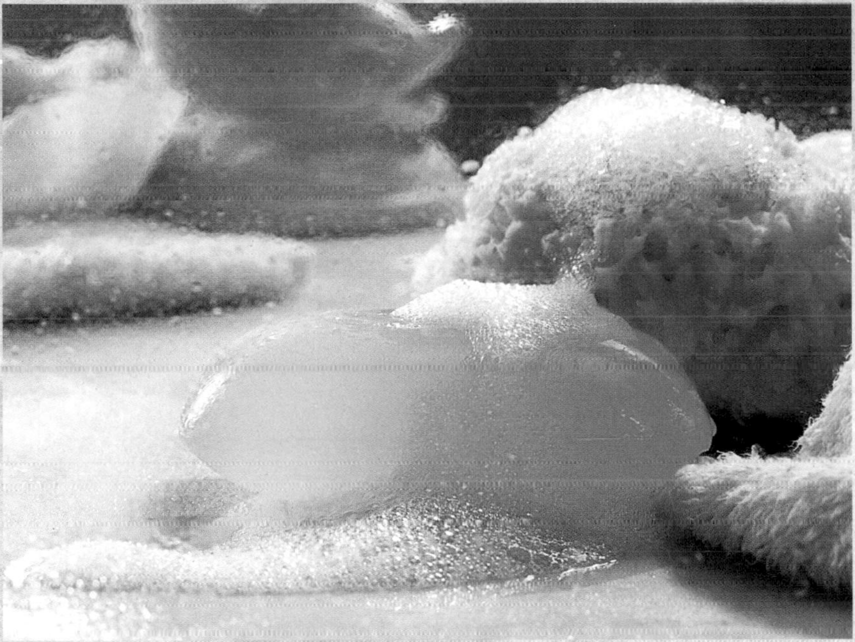

Stir lye flakes into cold water until dissolved. When fat is lukewarm, pour in lye, stirring to thicken. Add lanolin, glycerine, and essential oils, beating vigorously to disperse evenly. Pour into shaving mug and previously prepared and greased moulds. (Cardboard frozen orange juice containers are about the right size.) Recipe yields 12 ounces of hard bar soap and 1½ cups of liquid soap.

it could set you back as much as $2,400. Not to repine, however, because a good brush should last for twenty years or more. This could work out to around $120 a year. Which makes daily use of the most expensive shaving brush in the world a comparatively affordable pleasure.

The Ozone Layer

Until 1978, chlorofluorocarbons, also called freons, were the aerosol can propellant of choice. But fears that they act on ozone molecules with potentially devastating consequences for life on the planet led the U.S. government to strictly limit use of these compounds. In compliance with this federal ban, manufacturers substituted hydrocarbons and carbon dioxide in most aerosol products. So shavers need no longer feel guilty that they're doing their part every day to tear a bigger hole in the ozone.

Aftershave

Two thousand years before the birth of Christ, the Babylonian ruler Hammurabi decreed that

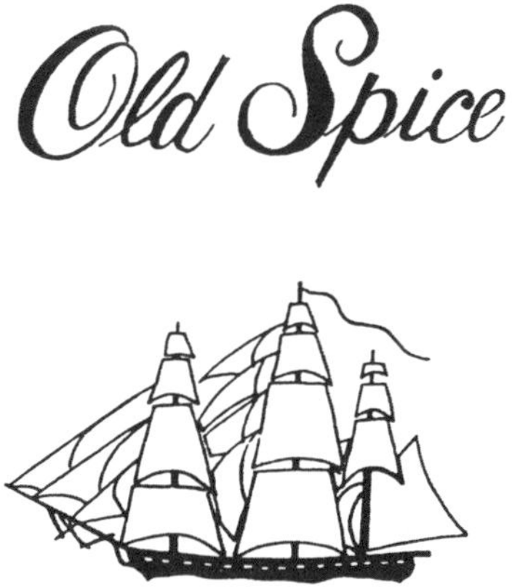

everyone in his kingdom should wash in perfume. Half a millennium later, Assyrian warriors curled their beards and anointed them with scented oils. On the threshold of the twenty-first century, American men prefer soap and water for their ablutions and are mostly clean-shaven, but we still want to smell good.

Aftershave should not only smell good, it should feel good too. If a man is shaving right, it will. If he's shaving wrong, it will feel like a colony of fire ants on his jaw. Tastes do differ, but this is not how most men want to start the day.

An aftershave feels good because it contains a little alcohol. The alcohol that stings on new nicks also cools the skin. One of the newer developments in men's cosmetics is aftershave lotion, which moisturizes and smooths the skin. Unlike cologne, which is designed to linger, the scent in aftershave performs only for a short time.

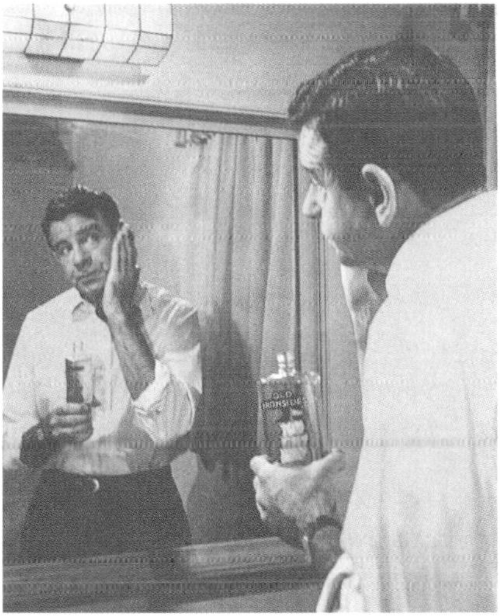

Above: Old Ironsides—Walter Matthau's aftershave of choice.

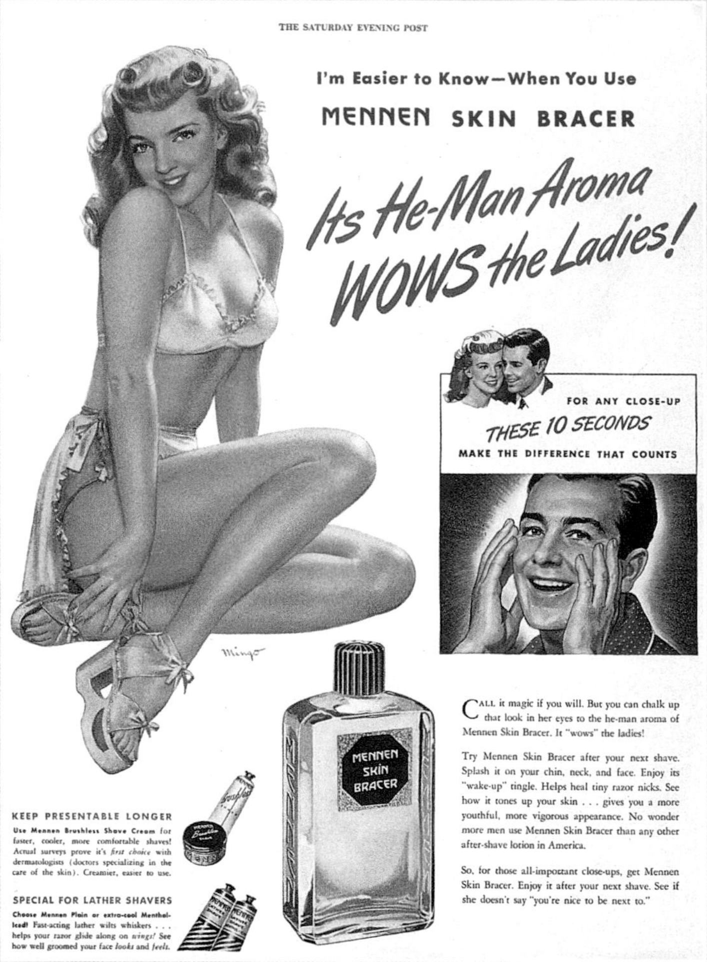
THE SATURDAY EVENING POST
I'm Easier to Know—When You Use
MENNEN SKIN BRACER
Its He-Man Aroma WOWS the Ladies!
FOR ANY CLOSE-UP
THESE 10 SECONDS
MAKE THE DIFFERENCE THAT COUNTS
Mingo
MENNEN SKIN BRACER
CALL it magic if you will. But you can chalk up that look in her eyes to the he-man aroma of Mennen Skin Bracer. It "wows" the ladies!
Try Mennen Skin Bracer after your next shave. Splash it on your chin, neck, and face. Enjoy its "wake-up" tingle. Helps heal tiny razor nicks. See how it tones up your skin . . . gives you a more youthful, more vigorous appearance. No wonder more men use Mennen Skin Bracer than any other after-shave lotion in America.
So, for those all-important close-ups, get Mennen Skin Bracer. Enjoy it after your next shave. See if she doesn't say "you're nice to be next to."
KEEP PRESENTABLE LONGER
Use Mennen Brushless Shave Cream for faster, cooler, more comfortable shaves! Actual surveys prove it's first choice with dermatologists (doctors specializing in the care of the skin). Creamier, easier to use.
SPECIAL FOR LATHER SHAVERS
Choose Mennen Plain or extra-cool Menthol-Iced! Fast-acting lather wilts whiskers . . . helps your razor glide along on wings! See how well groomed your face looks and feels.

"The Rules"

1. A man's aftershave should not have more personality than he does.

2. Even a used car salesman should use an aftershave without a hard sell.

3. The morning kiss should leave just enough aftershave lingering to remind her of him; but it should be gone well before she sees him at the end of the day. Otherwise it's a distraction and a nuisance.

4. A lingering aftershave that smells good on the woman it touches is a very good sign of compatibility.

5. Like a woman's perfume, a man's aftershave should fit with his chemistry, his personality, and his lifestyle. There are only a very few scents that will suit any one man. One is not too few.

6. It takes time to find the right aftershave, and once the few scents are discovered, they deserve fidelity. It's the only way to make them yours.

7. When a child smells a certain perfume, the child, no matter how much time has passed, will think of his or her mother. And when a child notices the faint trace of a certain aftershave, it should likewise evoke memories of Dad.

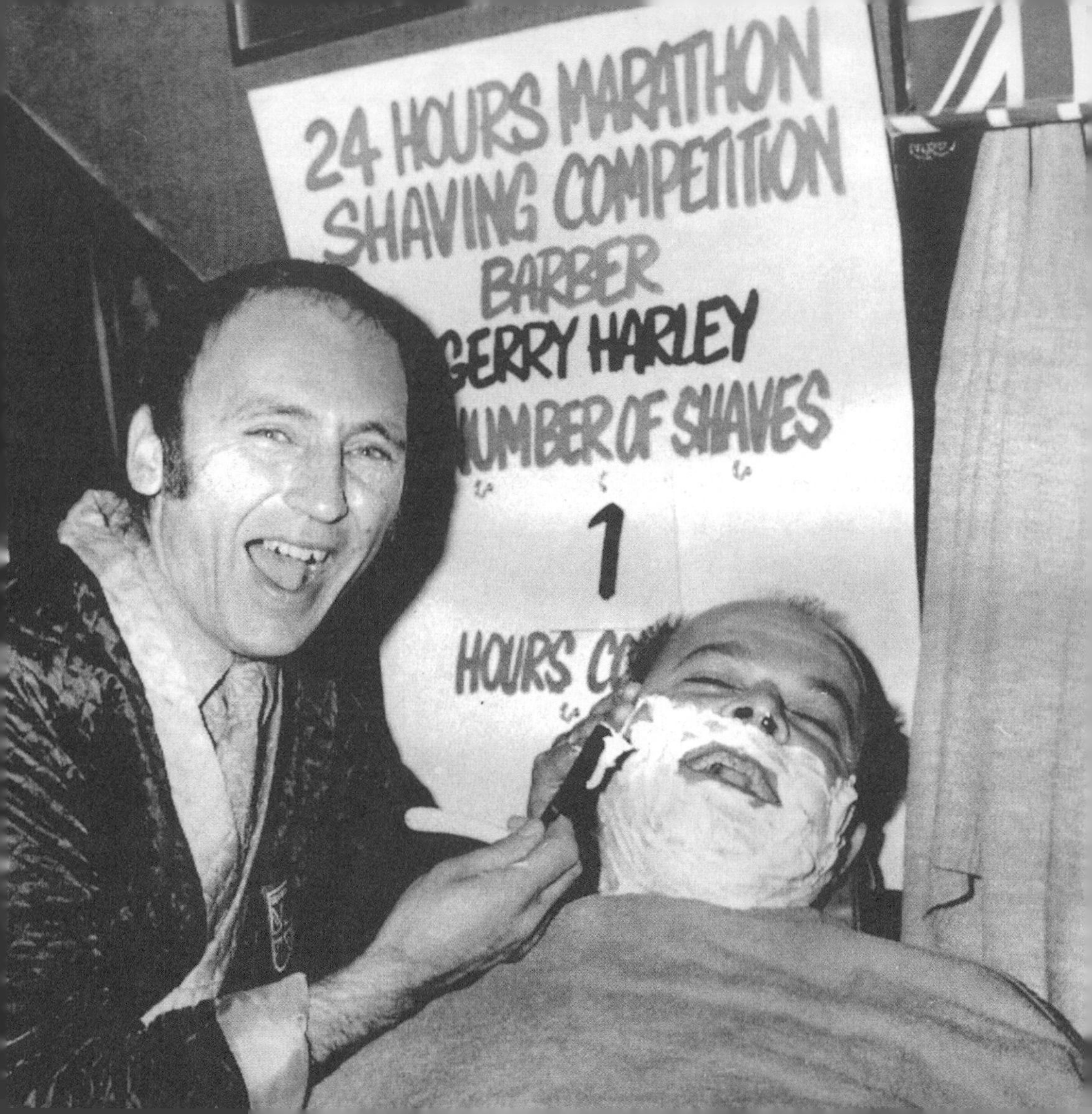

24 HOURS MARATHON
SHAVING COMPETITION
BARBER
GERRY HARLEY
NUMBER OF SHAVES
1

Superlatives

The two fastest-shaving barbers in the world, according to the *Guinness Book of World Records,* are both English. In 1984, Mr. Gerry Harley shaved 235 men in an hour using a straight razor. Only 1 man was nicked. Four years later, Mr. Denny Rowe was able to shave 1,994 men in the same lapse of time, averaging 1.8 seconds per customer. Mr. Rowe drew blood four times.

The longest beard ever recorded belonged to Hans Langseth of Norway. Born in 1846, he emigrated to the United States, where he died in 1927, leaving behind seventeen and a half feet of beard. Curiously, his heirs waited forty years to donate the beard to the Smithsonian Institution.

The biggest mustache in the world must be the one on the equestrian

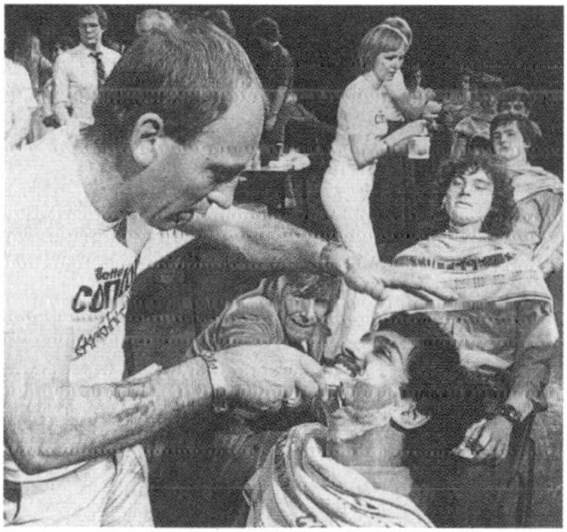

Left and above: We learn by doing. Harley, the "Lightning Barber," shaved 80 chins in an hour in 1970; he was up to 203 by 1979.

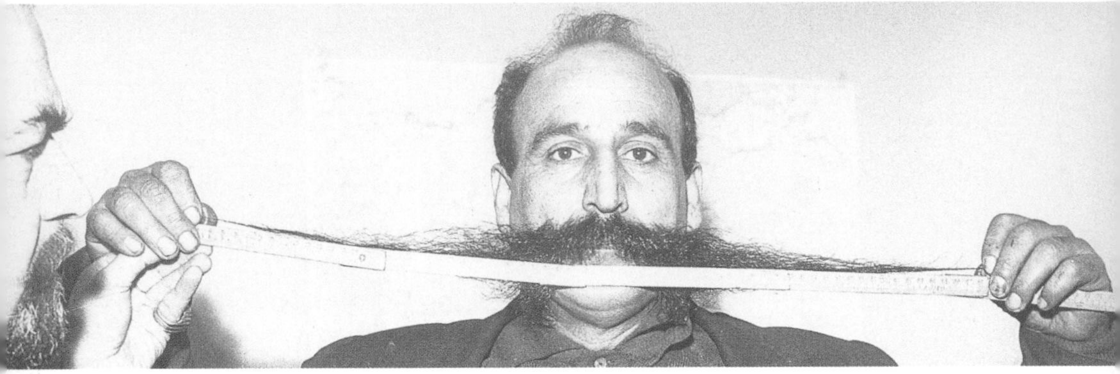

Above: In January 1964, Recep Dogruer of Turkey claimed to have the longest mustache in the world—a mere 68 inches.

statue of Vittorio Emmanuel II on the Altar of the Nation in Rome. The king's colossal white marble mustache measures three meters long. The longest mustache on a living human being belongs to Mr. Birger Pellas of Malmö, Sweden, who has not shaved his upper lip since 1973. In the mid-1990s, he had a ten-foot mustache to show for his forbearance.

The oddest death by a beard of extraordinary length befell Hans Steininger, who was chief magistrate of Braunau, Austria, in the 1500s, an age when beards were fiercely admired. Steininger's beard was eight feet nine inches long and had to be wrapped around his neck and tucked up across his chest when he walked around. On his way to a council meeting on September 28, 1567, the beard came undone. Steininger tripped over the end of it and fell down a flight of stairs to his death.

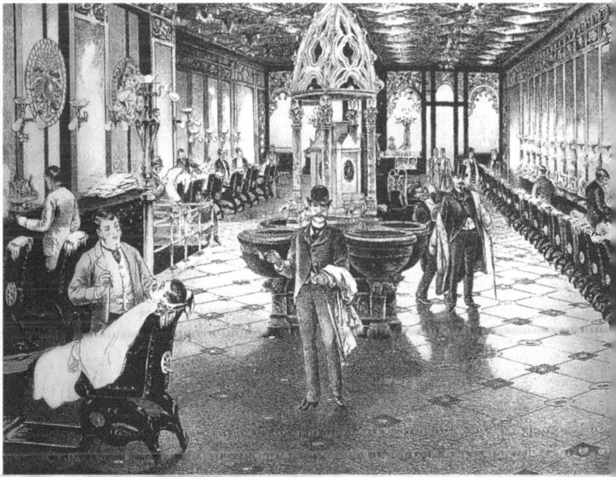

John M. Todd operated a barbershop in Portland, Maine, from 1845 to 1905 and his dauntingly entitled autobiography, *Sixty-two Years in a Barbershop*, relates some of the tonsorial records of his day:

Luke V. Whalen, the only official minute barber in the city, swears . . . that he lathered and shaved a man over twice in just one minute.

George N. Rich says he has got the figures to show that he shaved ninety men in one day.

D. C. Hutchins, the magician barber, often shaves a man a minute by way of recreation.

J. N. Pooler has removed the hair from the faces of eleven men in one hour.

George W. Damm, with a boy to help him lather, once shaved seventeen men in twenty minutes.

J. C. Moxcey has been plastering the lather on the human face forty-five years, and it is estimated that Mr. Moxcey and the razor have traveled in the aggregate over seven hundred and eighteen miles over human faces. In his younger years no more alert barber stood by the mug.

Shaving and the Movies

Everyone has a favorite razor scene from the movies: Michael Caine as a murderous transvestite surprising poor Angie Dickinson in the elevator in *Dressed to Kill;* Marlon Brando, oddly dressed as an old woman at times, getting what he deserves in *The Missouri Breaks.* Early in his career, Martin Scorsese made a short called *The Big Shave* in which a young man shaves himself again and again until he cuts his own throat. (The Library of Congress cross-references it under Shaving, Self-mutilation, and Comedy.)

No one who's seen *Le Chien*

Right: Cary Grant in *North by Northwest*

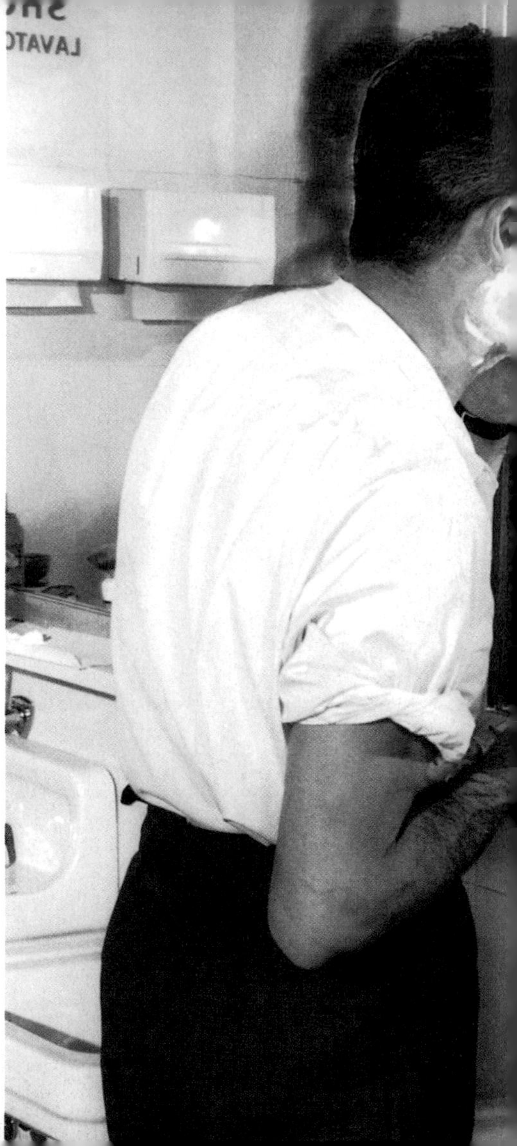

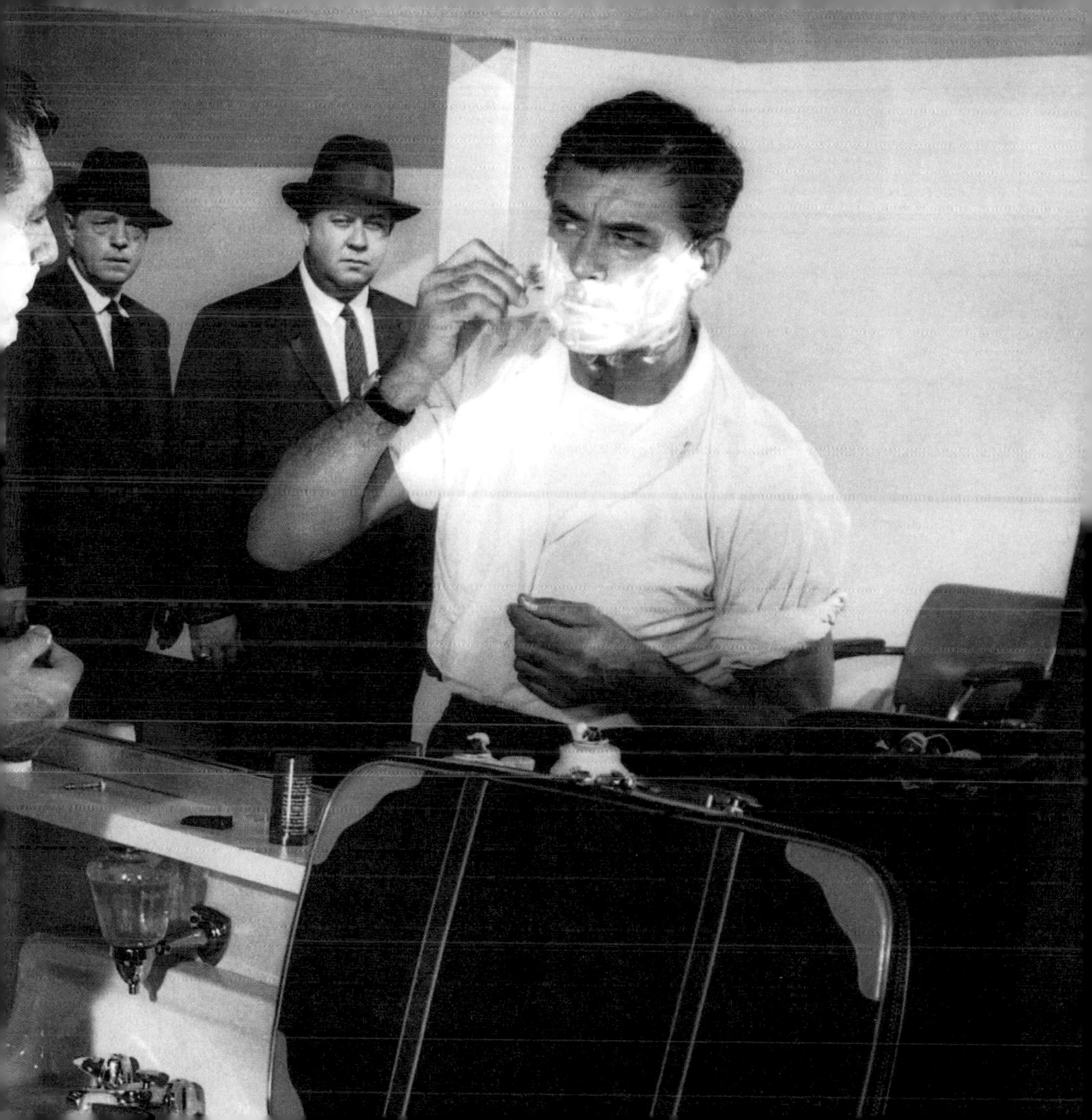

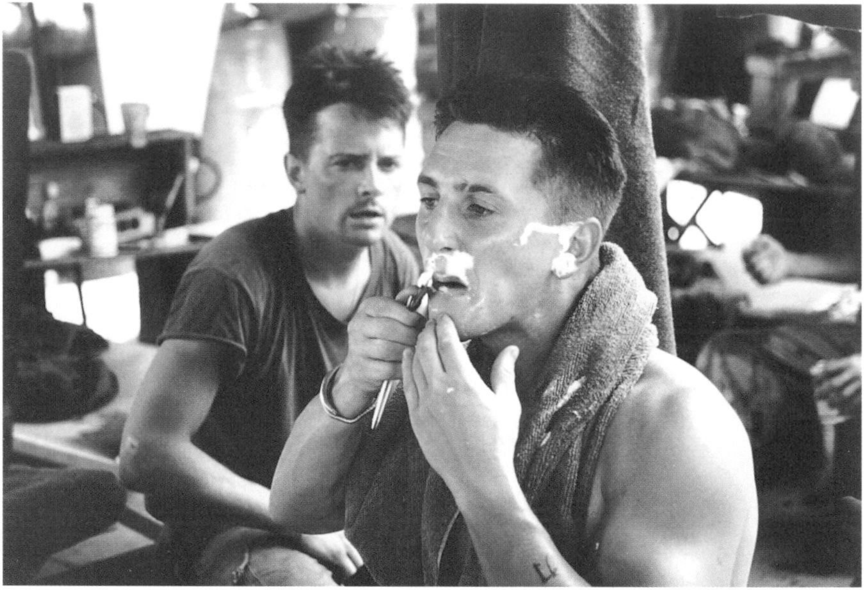

Above: Sean Penn shaves while Michael J. Fox looks on in *Casualties of War.*

Andalou will forget the scene that caused a riot in 1934 and still has the power to shock. From the script: "Once upon a time, a balcony was in the dark. Indoors a man was whetting his razor. He looked up through the window at the sky and saw a fleecy cloud drawing near to the full moon. Then a young girl's head with staring eyes. Now the fleecy cloud passes over the moon. And the razor blade passes through the girl's eye, slicing it in two."

In *North by Northwest,* Cary Grant, running for his life, has understandably not thought to bring his toilet kit with him and has to make do. One of the items he's confronted with is a tiny travel razor, about as big as a Barbie doll's arm. His look of perplexed annoyance deserves a place of its own on Mt. Rushmore.

In the 1950s, the electric razor was coming into its own. It had

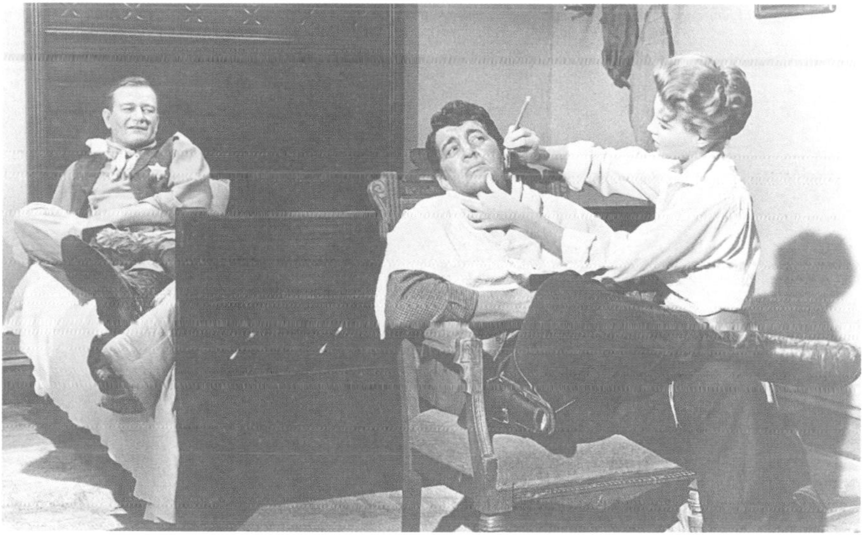

Above: In *Rio Bravo,* a reformed card shark with a steady hand (Angie Dickinson) shaves a reformed drunk with the shakes (Dean Martin), while John Wayne supervises.

Ever since 1910 the Gillette Company has used many a popular athlete to promote its products. The list of ball players who shaved on camera for Gillette reads like an all-star roster: Bob Feller, Warren Spahn, Roy Campanella, Willie Mays, Maury Wills, Pee Wee Reese, Elston Howard. So many that it became baseball folklore that a player really hadn't made it out of the bush leagues if he hadn't been signed by Gillette.

The owners of various ball clubs have had a lot to say about the hairstyles and facial hair of their players over the years. New York Yankees owner George Steinbrenner is notoriously dictatorial when it comes to the personal grooming of his players. In the 1970s, when many American men wore their hair long and affected beards, side-burns, and mustaches, he wanted his team to look and behave like the teams of the 1950s. Left fielder Lou Piniella was once called into Steinbrenner's office to defend the length of his hair. Using the Bible as his defense, Piniella told his boss that Jesus had long hair too. To which Steinbrenner replied, "Oh yeah? Well, when you can walk on water, I'll let you have long hair. Now, go get a haircut."

Other ball clubs were more relaxed. In the same decade that Steinbrenner was giving his players boot camp advice on how to look sharp and be sharp, Oakland

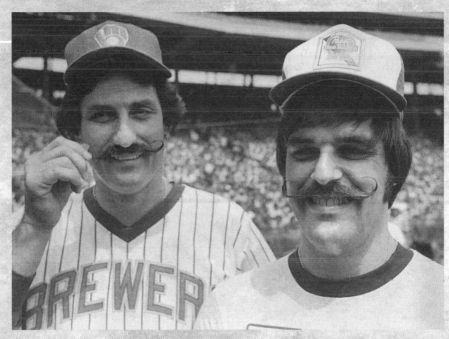

Above: Six hundred men entered a statewide handlebar mustache competition. The winner, Jerry Mlodzik, is pictured here with Milwaukee Brewers pitcher Rollie Fingers in August 1982.

Athletics management offered players bonuses to grow facial hair, the better to resemble their counterparts of the 1920s. Rollie Fingers is remembered as much for the extravagant handlebar mustache that became his trademark as he is for his great pitching.

been around since the late 1930s, but smaller batteries, and the progress of plastic technology, allowed for brightly colored, cordless models. Throughout the decade, the razor was the gadget emblem of the modern man. Anthony Quinn used one in *The Long Wait;* James Stewart had his leg in a cast but could shave himself without budging from his wheelchair in *Rear Window;* and that's how Humphrey Bogart shaves in *Sabrina.*

BURMA SHAVE

Before shaving foam with aloe, before gel with vitamin E, before Interstate 80 and Interstate 295, there was Burma-Shave. Burma-Shave's advertising campaign for its brushless shaving cream may not have been *the* most successful ever conducted, but it's certainly one of the most affectionately remembered. From 1926 to 1963, its quintets of rhyming signs sprouted along American roadsides, and gave bored children, riding in the backseat on endless car trips, a reason to live.

Allan Odell, the inventor's son (and the company's resident poet), came up with the idea of rhyming signs and placed the first ones on U.S. 65, near Lakeville, Minnesota:

HALF A POUND
FOR
HALF A DOLLAR
SPREAD ON THIN
ABOVE THE COLLAR
BURMA-SHAVE

More followed:

HE HAD THE RING
HE HAD THE FLAT
BUT SHE FELT HIS
CHIN
AND THAT
WAS THAT
BURMA-SHAVE

HE PLAYED
A SAX
HAD NO B.O.
BUT HIS WHISKERS
SCRATCHED
SO SHE LET HIM GO
BURMA-SHAVE

TO GET
AWAY FROM
HAIRY APES
LADIES JUMP FROM
FIRE ESCAPES
BURMA-SHAVE

It saved time:

EVERY SHAVER
NOW CAN SNORE
SIX MORE MINUTES
THAN BEFORE
BURMA-SHAVE

It taught history:

HENRY THE EIGHTH
SURE HAD
TROUBLE
SHORT-TERM WIVES
LONG-TERM STUBBLE
BURMA-SHAVE

It kept up with the times:

FREE
FREE
A TRIP TO MARS
FOR 900
EMPTY JARS
BURMA-SHAVE

And it recognized the human condition:

WITHIN THIS VALE
OF TOIL
AND SIN
YOUR HEAD GROWS
BALD
BUT NOT YOUR CHIN
BURMA-SHAVE

Truth in advertising, 1930s style, brought to motorists by Burma-Shave.

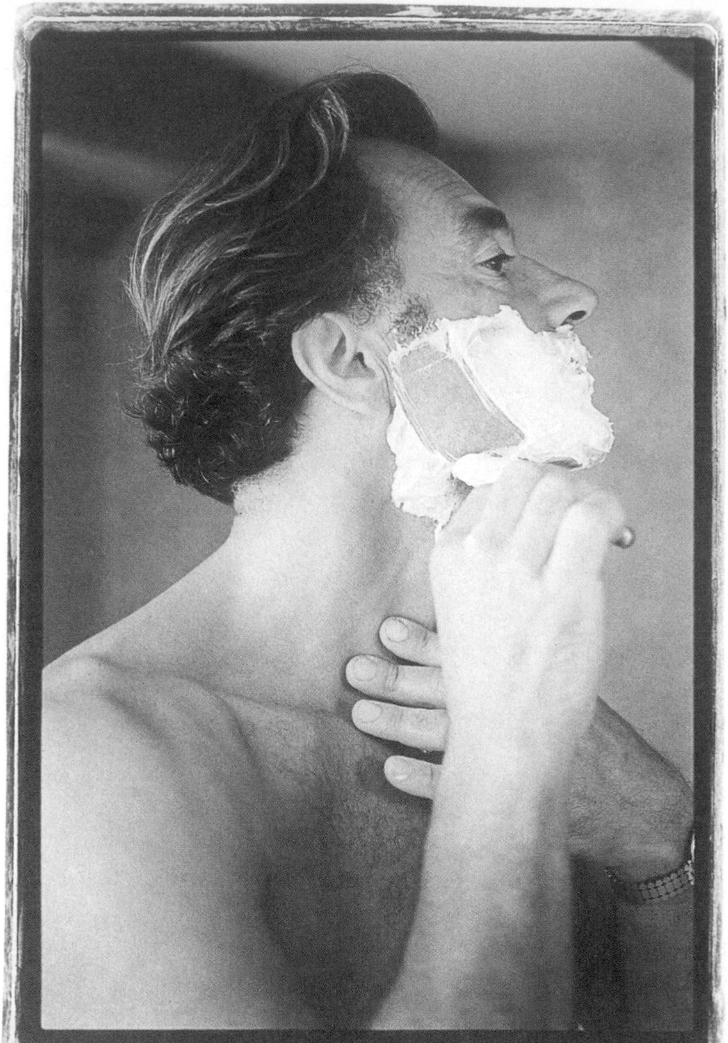

My Father Shaves with Occam's Razor

Entities must not be
unnecessarily multiplied.

William of Occam

The simplest of answers
is preferred. Explanations
of the unknown should first
be sought in what is near.

So with love and poetry;
what we can't make out
we seek in the seen,
ice, fire, stone, steam.

Shaving away another day
I recall watching my father—
flecks, specks of soap.
Ooo, blood! Such longing.

Where has he gone? Not
cloudward, to rise and fall
on wires taut as harp string—
and what parent ever
was consigned to fire
ever and ever?—but here,
a rectangle on the wall,
every morning mirror,

darkness between lips,
a song, this very voice,
the blinding light of eyes.
Each night he grows in me,

appears at dawn at the end
of dream, his hand moving
in billows of steam.
And just like him I bleed.

David Citino

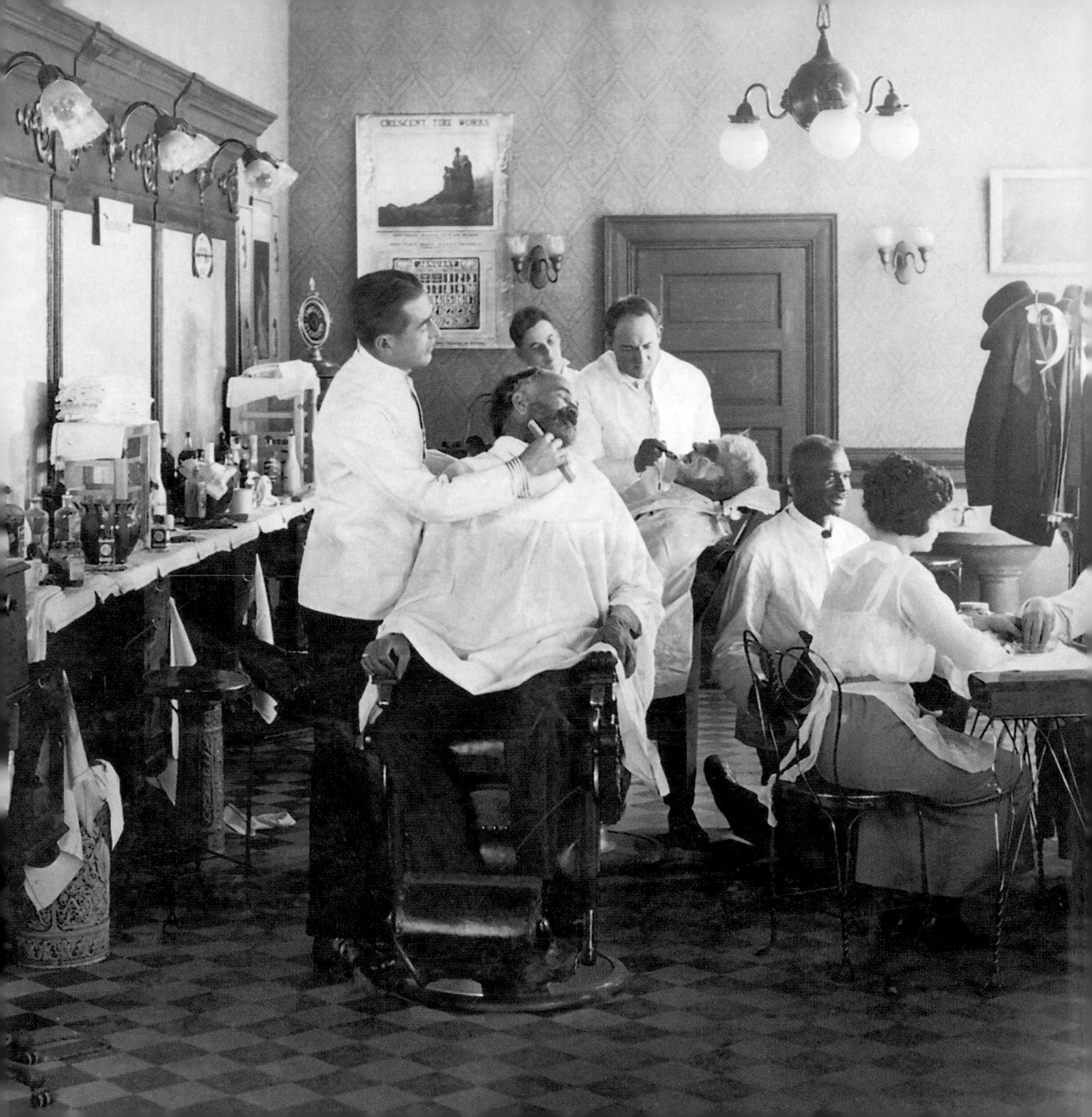
CRESCENT TIRE WORKS

ACKNOWLEDGMENTS

Many friends and acquaintances have shared their knowledge and experience of shaving customs and beard-care with me. I owe special thanks to Jane Sarnoff and James Pinfold.

I am also indebted to: Pete Duffey of the Hair Shoppe, Daphne Howland, Ethan Howland, John Howland, Sam Berlind, Kevin Bubriskie, John Spritz, John David Werner, Dr. Nancy Egan, Dr. Peter Evans, Peter De Staebler, Vance Muse, Sara Dickey, José Ribas, Marc Libby, Rick Jones of Gentlemen's Choice (Boston), Arthur Marks of Stoddards (Boston), Ruth Abraham Fisher, Hoyt Rogers, Bruce Balboni, Latif Ndiaye, Michael Weber, Paul Heroux, Scott Goldberg, Alan Long, Margaret Burchenal, Steve Caton, Ruth Tracy, Mokha Laghet, Dan Whitman, Sim Smiley, and Peter Girouard of the Colonial Barber Shop in Portland, Maine.

The reference staffs at Curtis Memorial Library, the Bowdoin College Library, and the Fragrance Foundation were unfailingly helpful.

Phillip L. Krumholz's books and articles on barber supplies and shaving equipment have answered questions I didn't know people asked.

Without the diligence and imagination of my editor, Tricia Boczkowski, and the resourcefulness of photo researcher Alexandra Truitt, this would have been a poorer book. Without the original idea and encouragement of Amy Gash, there would have been no book at all.

The credit is theirs; the errors my own.

PHOTOGRAPHY AND ILLUSTRATION CREDITS

Every effort has been made to account for and credit the copyright owners of the archival photographs, illustrations, and text included in this book. Any inadvertent omissions should be brought to the attention of the author, care of the publisher. All brands and product names are trademarks or registered trademarks of their respective companies.

Pages 1, 3, Mary Evans Picture Library; pages 6–7, Henri Cartier-Bresson/Magnum Photos; page 8, Mary Evans Picture Library; page 9, Mary Evans Picture Library; page 11, Daily Mirror/Corbis-Bettmann; page 12, Hulton Getty/Liaison Agency; page 13, James Faris; page 14, Hulton Getty/Liaison Agency; page 17, DC Comics/Photofest; page 18, Corbis; page 20, Mary Evans Picture Library; page 22, Corbis-Bettmann; page 24, Mary Evans Picture Library; page 26, Christie's Images; page 27, The Granger Collection, New York; page 28, Mary Evans Picture Library; page 29, The Granger Collection, New York; page 30, The Granger Collection, New York; page 31, Mary Evans Picture Library; page 32, published courtesy of the Fruitlands Museums, Harvard, Massachusetts; page 33, The Granger Collection, New York; page 34 (*both*), The Granger Collection, New York; page 35 (*both*), The Granger Collection, New York; page 36, Corbis-Bettmann; page 37, Corbis-Bettmann; page 38, UPI/Corbis-Bettmann; page 39, © Richard Vogel/Gamma Liaison; page 40, Christie's Images/SuperStock; page 41, Christie's Images; page 44, SuperStock; page 45, © Anthony Edgeworth/The Stock Market; page 47, Christie's Images; page 48, The Advertising Archives; page 51, Photofest; page 52, UPI/Corbis-Bettmann; page 55, © Brad Trent; page 56, UPI/Corbis-Bettmann; page 57, Gamma Liaison; page 58, UPI/Corbis-Bettmann; page 59, Mary Evans Picture Library; page 60, The Granger Collection, New York; page 61, SuperStock; page 62, UPI/Corbis-Bettmann; page 63, Baldwin H. Ward/Corbis-Bettmann; page 67, Mary Evans Picture Library; page 68, Corbis-Bettmann; page 69, Corbis-Bettmann; page 70, Corbis-Bettmann; page 71, Corbis-Bettmann; page 72, Corbis-Bettmann; page 73, Corbis-Bettmann; page 75, Archive Photos; page 76, Andrew Eccles/Outline; page 77, Camera Press, Ltd./Archive Photos; page 78, Photofest; page 79, © Gerard Vandystadt/Allsport; page 80, SuperStock; page 82, from *Modern Textbook on Barbering* published by Vaughn Barber Schools; page 83, SuperStock; pages 84–85, Petrified Collection/The Image Bank; page 87, Corbis-Bettmann; page 88, SuperStock; page 90, Mary Evans Picture Library; page 91, Reuters/Corbis-Bettmann; page 92, Corbis-Bettmann; page 95, UPI/Corbis-Bettmann; page 96 (*top*), © Brad Trent; page 96 (*bottom*), Corbis-Bettmann; page 97 (*top*), Corbis-Bettmann; page 97 (*bottom*), Mary Evans Picture Library; page 98, Christie's Images; page 99 (*left*), Christie's Images; page 99 (*right*), © Brad Trent; page 100 (*top*), Christie's Images; page 100 (*bottom*), Stock Montage/SuperStock; page 101 (*top*), Corbis-

Bettmann; page 101 (*bottom*), The Granger Collection, New York; page 102, Photofest; page 103 (*top left*), Corbis-Bettmann; page 103 (*bottom left*), Mary Evans Picture Library; page 103 (*right*), courtesy of The Gillette Company; page 104, Mary Evans Picture Library; page 105 (*both*), UPI/Corbis-Bettmann; page 106 (*top*), The Advertising Archives; page 106 (*bottom*), UPI/Corbis-Bettmann; page 107, UPI/Corbis-Bettmann; page 108 (*left*), Hulton Getty/Liaison Agency; page 108 (*right*), Gamma Liaison; page 109, © Jed Jacobsohn/Allsport; page 110, © Zigy Kaluzny/Gamma Liaison; page 111, Mary Evans Picture Library; pages 112–113, © Zigy Kaluzny/Gamma Liaison; page 115, © Zigy Kaluzny/Gamma Liaison; page 116, by permission of the makers of Barbasol® shave cream; page 117, Brown Brothers; page 118, Mary Evans Picture Library; page 119, Graphic House/Corbis Bettmann; page 121, The Advertising Archives; page 122, Gamma Liaison; page 124, The Advertising Archives; page 125, © Rosemary Weller/Tony Stone Images; page 126, © Brad Trent; page 127, Archive Photos; pages 128–129, Archive Photos; page 131, The Advertising Archives; page 132, The Advertising Archives; page 133, PhotoDisc; page 134, Corbis-Bettmann; page 135, © Garry Gay/The Image Bank; page 137, © Luc Hautecoeur/Tony Stone Images; page 138, Old Spice® is a registered trademark of Procter & Gamble, and is used with permission; page 139, Photofest; page 140, The Advertising Archives; page 142, UPI/Corbis-Bettmann; page 143, UPI/Corbis-Bettmann; page 144, Express Newspapers/Archive Photos; page 145, Corbis-Bettmann; pages 146–147, The Kobal Collection; page 148, Photofest; page 149, The Kobal Collection; page 151, UPI/Corbis-Bettmann; pages 152-153, Burma-Shave® is a registered trademark of the American Safety Razor Co.; page 154, © Butch Martin/The Image Bank; page 156, The Granger Collection, New York; page 160, The Advertising Archives.

TEXT CREDITS

Page 69, from *Tossing and Turning* by John Updike. Copyright © 1970 by John Updike. Reprinted by permission of Alfred A. Knopf, Inc.; pages 86, 89–90, from *History of Shaving and Razors* by Phillip L. Krumholz. Copyright © 1987 by Phillip L. Krumholz, P.O. Box 4050, Bartonville, IL 61607. Reprinted by permission of the author; pages 90-92, from *Justine* by Lawrence Durrell. Copyright © 1957 by Lawrence Durrell. Graciously reprinted by permission of the Estate of Lawrence Durrell; pages 92–93, from "My Life on the Edge" by Cal Fussman. Copyright © 1991 by Cal Fussman. Originally published in *GQ*. Reprinted by permission of the author; pages 93–94, excerpted from "By the Hair of Your Chinny Chin Chin" by Richard Brookhiser. Reprinted by permission of FORBES FYI Magazine. Copyright © Forbes Inc., 1996; pages 116–117, from *Babbitt* by Sinclair Lewis. Copyright © 1922 by Harcourt Brace & Co. and renewed 1950 by Sinclair Lewis, Preprinted by permission of the publisher; page 126, "The Razor" by Marvin Solomon. Copyright © 1995 by The Modern Poetry Association. Originally published in POETRY. Reprinted by permission of the editor of POETRY; page 155, "My Father Shaves with Occam's Razor" by David Citino. Copyright © 1993 by The Modern Poetry Association. Originally published in POETRY. Reprinted by permission of the editor of POETRY.

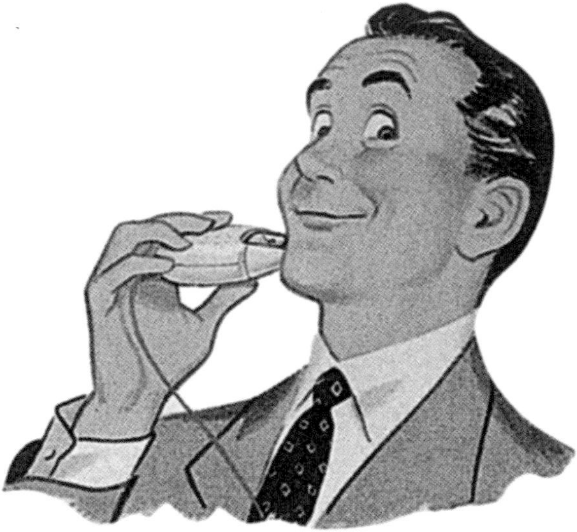